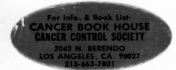

For Info. & Book List-
CANCER BOOK HOUSE
CANCER CONTROL SOCIETY
2043 N. BERENDO
LOS ANGELES, CA. 90027
213-663-7801

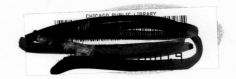

CHICAGO PUBLIC LIBRARY

D1261384

HOW TO
CONQUER
ARTHRITIS

Other Books by John H. Tobe

GROWING FLOWERS
EAT RIGHT AND BE HEALTHY
ROMANCE IN THE GARDEN
VIRILITY, STAMINA THROUGH ENZYMES
GARDEN GLIMPSES
SPROUTS — ELIXIR OF LIFE
BANISH BACKACHE
PROVEN HERBAL REMEDIES
ASPIRIN — MONSTER IN DISGUISE
MILK — FRIEND OR FIEND?
THE "NO-COOK" BOOK
LET'S MAKE OUR OWN WINES AND BEERS
SALT AND YOUR HEALTH
"BONSAI" — DWARF POTTED TREES
GUIDEPOSTS TO HEALTH
HUNZA: ADVENTURES IN A LAND OF PARADISE
YOUR PROSTATE
MARGARINE AND YOUR HEART ATTACK
I FOUND SHANGRI-LA
SECURITY FROM FIVE ACRES
THE GOLDEN TREASURY OF NATURAL HEALTH
CATARACT, GLAUCOMA AND OTHER EYE DISORDERS
HOW TO PREVENT AND GAIN REMISSION FROM CANCER

HOW TO CONQUER ARTHRITIS

by John H. Tobe

Printed and Published in Canada by

PROVOKER PRESS
ST. CATHARINES, ONT.
1976

© COPYRIGHT, CANADA, 1976

By JOHN H. TOBE, St. Catharines, Ont.,

All rights reserved — no part of this book may be reproduced in any form without permission in writing from the publisher, except by a reviewer who wishes to quote brief passages in connection with a review written for inclusion in a magazine or newspaper.

Printed in Canada

TABLE OF CONTENTS

Chapter   **Page**

1.	Is There An Arthritis Philosophy Or Psychology? .	1
2.	The Medical Profession's Pet	5
3.	Everybody's Disease	17
4.	Early Detection Means Earlier Crippling	23
5.	Main Causes Of Arthritis	31
6.	An Enzyme Deficiency Disease	37
7.	Essential Unsaturated Fatty Acids	41
8.	Vitamin D	45
9.	Metabolism Of Calcium And Phosphorus	51
10.	Bread And Other Wheat Products	57
11.	Tea For Two	63
12.	Frozen Foods And Vitamin K	67
13.	Arthritis And Your Emotions	71
14.	Relief Of Pain	77
15.	The Medical Profession's Answer	83
16.	Artificial Joints	91
17.	Chiropractors And Arthritis	103
18.	Sex And Arthritis	111
19.	Aspirin	115
20.	Fasting As A Treatment For Arthritis	123
21.	Mineral Baths, Spas And Climatic Changes	129

22. Cod Liver Oil And Arthritis 137
23. Cider Vinegar And Honey 143
24. Various Treatments For Arthritis 153
25. New Drugs 173
26. Raw Food 181
27. Only Nature Can Cure 201
28. Questions And Answers 209

INTRODUCTION

In my writing I always feel it necessary to specify most emphatically that I am not a healer of any kind. I am a researcher, an investigator, an observer and a writer, who is seriously interested in health in all its phases.

As I have repeatedly stated, if I felt that the use of drugs, radium, surgery, abracadabra, mumbo-jumbo or witch-doctoring in any form whatsoever would bring health to people, I would be totally in favor of it. However, a lifetime of investigation has proven to me, without a shadow of doubt, that the way to health lies in following natural biological law which is the way animals live in their native habitat. I believe that was the way it was intended and that is the way it is. I am, of course, referring to a proper raw food diet and proper living habits.

I do want to make it clear and to the point that I am a reporter and when I hear of a method or means that has brought health to someone, if it is worth mentioning, I mention it. I do not set myself up as any supreme authority. I am a truth seeker on health matters . . . in fact, all matters. Therefore, when I refer to and give data concerning various means of achieving a cure, good health or easing suffering, it does not mean that I advise or endorse the method or form of treatment. (This statement is more or less what is called a disclaimer.)

I don't want to be accused of recommending, suggesting or advising 'kooky' cures, yet I don't want to ignore something that can bring relief to suffering mankind.

CHAPTER 1

IS THERE AN ARTHRITIS PHILOSOPHY
OR PSYCHOLOGY?

After observing, studying and interviewing arthritics or arthritis sufferers for at least 20 years, I sometimes have to ask myself the question which is the title of this chapter, "Is there an arthritis philosophy or psychology?" That is, is there an arthritis way of life?

Many years ago I read a story about a plain ordinary man who had known little of greatness or importance or the V.I.P. treatment. He led a very dull and uninteresting life until one day he was accidentally hurt at his job. His injuries necessitated a short period in the hospital and then crutches. He couldn't drive his car so he had to take the bus to work and, because he was crippled, the bus driver used to pull up close to the curb and get out and help him on or off the bus. People would get up to give him a seat and everyone was solicitous and concerned about him. Suddenly he found that he was a somebody, he was important and he was enjoying something he had never had before in his whole life. So it is not hard to understand why he was a long, long time getting over his injury.

I recall the case of a very ordinary, rather dull gentleman, who sold a little bit of insurance in the little town where I lived for 40 years. I don't think he made much

1

money but he managed to keep body and soul together. Eventually he developed arthritis and for a time it became so bad he had to use crutches to get around. Suddenly his mediocre business zoomed. It seems that everyone wanted to help this poor crippled fellow. Well, I can assure you that those crutches remained part and parcel of his life.

I knew this man very well and I learned that he could walk without the crutches . . . but only when he thought he was not being observed. He drove his car and he handled it to perfection, but he would hobble to and from the car. Out of the car he was crippled but in it he was perfectly all right.

I talk to many men and women who are afflicted with arthritis and I say, "You don't have to suffer from arthritis. I can show you how you can defeat the condition and regain your normal health and mobility."

Occasionally some folks take me up on this statement and I show them how they can get rid of their arthritis by changing their way of life and their diet . . . and they can get rid of their arthritis, if they really want to. However, I have learned that there are many victims of arthritis who prefer the pain to losing the many advantages gained by being crippled with this disease. Now I am not saying this is the rule — I am just reporting what I have observed.

Because of the condition they are the object of grave concern by their loved ones and associates and are pleased with the solicitous attitude of everyone — everyone being so concerned and kind. They like the various pleasant treatments — and there are pleasant treatments; for example, massage. Then too, they like the number of special privileges they receive, such as being given consideration when they shop or seek a service. Because no one wants to see them stand and suffer a long time, people give them their place in line or a seat on the bus and are kind and attentive. At home, they usually manage to avoid dish washing, don't have to carry out the garbage and are not expected to perform any one of a

2

thousand other chores around the home. They do not have to accept responsibility — it is not expected of them. They are left alone at home where they can live in peace and quiet. No one will bother them because they don't want to see them suffer. There is also the binding effect it has upon loved ones and those who really care.

Yes, many patients actually need their arthritic pains to survive and if one were to remove their pains, their whole world would collapse around them. Then they would once again have to take their place in the mainstream of life . . . the rat race.

A medical researcher brought forth an interesting highlight on the subject of family dynamics in relation to patients suffering pain when he stated that the most common situation is that the family member with pain becomes isolated. "No one asks him or her to do anything so the remaining family form a separate group. The patient feels helpless because no one makes any demands, for if they do, he then has pain and this perpetuates the whole system."

Then this writer goes on to tell of the ways and means of handling these cases and we quote:

"We try to break that after he has been under treatment for several weeks. We will draw up a schedule, possibly for him just to go with the family to a hockey game, or show. And this is enforced rigorously. We try to bring them back into the social circle again. It is one of the most difficult things to do but the most rewarding for the patient."

This is referred to as 'behaviour modification therapy' and it is claimed that it has been found effective in the relief of chronic pain that has been unresponsive to traditional methods of treatment. This finding is from a group of McMaster University investigators.

Then there are those arthritic sufferers who suffer needlessly for only one reason and that is because they believe their physician, the Arthritis Foundation and other societies who tell them there is no known cause and no known cure. Rather than go elsewhere for help and try some other ways and means, they prefer to accept the word of their medical advisor. It is easier that way and, besides, they have complete confidence in their physician.

I feel that it is important to consider these aspects because I contend that arthritis can be conquered — but there is a big proviso here — provided the patient or victim wants to be helped or genuinely wants to lose his pain or his arthritis.

CHAPTER 2

THE MEDICAL PROFESSION'S PET

I suggest that arthritis is the medical profession's greatest sinecure. I suggest that arthritis is to the medical man what a money-printing machine is to the government. As long as the medical doctor has a few arthritic patients, he will not be short of money to keep him in luxury for the rest of his life.

As far as the medical man is concerned there is no known cause and no known cure, yet he keeps on prescribing, treating and taking money. Because you are in pain and are suffering, you demand treatment, so the doctor keeps trying out all his new drugs on you. In this way he pleases the pharmaceutical and drug corporations, too. However, it is an undeniable fact that these drugs cause other more serious complications which means that you will keep going back to the doctor for the rest of your life.

Arthritis is said to be one of the oldest diseases known to man, but strange to relate, it is unknown to all non-domesticated animals. Incidentally, man is the only animal who cooks his food and with cooked food comes arthritis. It is interesting to note that domesticated or zoo-raised animals are fed cooked, processed foods and are also subject to arthritis. It was a sad day when man learned how to fire his food, for it was then that arthritis was born.

Part of the medical profession's strategy for treating

5

arthritis is to teach the sufferer to live with the disease. It is undeniable that the medical doctor actually tries in many ways to make the arthritic's crippling, painful life more comfortable with his treatments, services and drugs. If you are in severe pain, he will take you into the hospital, give you the required drugs to make you more comfortable and see that you are given good attention. Then all you have to do is recover from the side effects of the drugs that were given to you to dull or lull the pain.

I came across what I consider to be very important information in a booklet written by Dr. Walter C. Alvarez, who was afflicted with rheumatoid arthritis. He wrote this booklet to provide help for his newspaper readers. I think it gives you the picture of arthritis and also tells you some interesting things about the methods of treatment used by the medical profession.

However, before I quote from this booklet let me give you some pertinent data on Dr. Alvarez. He is Emeritus Consultant in Medicine, Mayo Clinic, and Emeritus Professor of Medicine, University of Minnesota, Mayo Graduate School.

Dr. Alvarez is a member of 52 medical societies, also an honorary member of various medical societies including the Royal Society of Medicine of England, the Gastroenterologic Society of Paris, and the National Academy of Medicine of Spain.

He has been editor-in-chief of the American Journal of Digestive Diseases; of Gastroenterology; of GP; of Modern Medicine, and Geriatrics. He is the author of many hundreds of medical articles, innumerable editorials and many books.

I am giving you all of this data and the pedigree because I want you to know that this doctor is one of the high muck-a-mucks in the medical profession and that when he says something it is akin to 'word from on high.'

Now I will quote from Dr. Alvarez's booklet entitled, "Arthritis and Rheumatism":

The term 'Arthritis' is used to designate any one of several types of trouble in joints. The word arthritis has largely replaced the old word, 'rheumatism.'

What Causes Arthritis?

In our efforts to help people with arthritis, we doctors have always been much handicapped by the fact that, in most cases, we have only the vaguest idea of the cause. When one does not know the cause, one cannot work logically toward a cure. We suspect that in most cases the cause is some disturbance in body chemistry; in another it may be infection; in another it can be ageing or wearing out of the joint; in another it seems to be what is called an autoimmune reaction, in which the joint may have become allergic to the rest of the body.

What People Should Know Before They Start Trying to Get Help for Their Arthritis

It is good if a patient's doctor can tell what type of arthritis is present.

Fibrositis

Millions of persons who think they have arthritis really have the much milder fibrositis, which is one of the commonest diseases of man. It tends, at intervals, to keep bothering the person, sometimes from his childhood to his old age. Fortunately, it doesn't deform the joints; it rarely cripples the person, and it doesn't turn into anything serious. I have had it all my life and, so far, none of my joints has become deformed. I have had dozens of attacks in which, for a few days or several weeks or even several months, some of my joints were sore and a bit stiff. I never did anything about the trouble, and so far, the pain and stiffness have always gone away.

Whenever I have waked in the morning with a painful and stiff hip-joint or ankle-joint, I have made it a point to walk to work, and always, by the time I have gone a few blocks, I have been free of pain, and free of it for the rest of

7

the day. As my old friend, Dr. Philip Hench used to say, the person who has guts enough to keep moving his sore joints may get well, while the one who nurses the joint and does not use it much has trouble.

Here is a perfect example of the contention that I have been making for more than 20 years. What's the use of going to a doctor, paying him good money, accepting his drugs and having him put you in the hospital when he doesn't know his rump from his elbow? In simple terms, doctors cannot help themselves and they cannot help their own families, so how are they going to help you?

Note that he said, "I have had it all my life, and, so far, none of my joints has become deformed."

Sure, his joints haven't become deformed because he probably hasn't taken all those drugs he usually prescribes for his trusting, believing patients. However, there are hundreds of thousands of arthritis sufferers in the United States who have become deformed after undergoing treatment by medical doctors like Dr. Alvarez.

In this same booklet he describes the various forms of arthritis and I will list them for you here: fibrositis, bursitis, neuritis, senescent arthritis, rheumatoid arthritis, spondylitis, rheumatic fever, infectious arthritis, gout, arthritis with psoriasis, Heberden's nodes, sciatica, a 'slipped' or ruptured disc and psychogenic rheumatism. There you have it — all those conditions — and, by their own admission, *doctors do not know the cause nor can they offer you a cure.*

I wish I could have quoted the whole booklet but space does not allow. I have never read more inane, sheer nonsense than I found in the pages of this booklet by this great, famous and renowned physician.

On page 21 of this booklet it is stated: "Experts agree that there is no special diet that has any curative effect on arthritis."

I have maintained for years and I maintain today that 30

days on a properly balanced raw food diet would show you enough improvement to convince you that a proper way of life is the answer to arthritis in its various forms . . . just as it is to most diseases that afflict mankind. Try a raw food diet for 30 days and you will quickly learn that the medical profession is deliberately lying.

You may ask, "Why are they deliberately lying?"

My answer is simple, "They must know that a raw food diet works and they don't want to lose 25,000,000 patients. So they keep on perpetuating the lie that there is no known cause and there is no known cure and that diet doesn't work."

You may think to yourself, "What am I to believe?"

To find the answer to that question, just try a 30-day diet of raw food. You will not starve and you will not harm yourself, because for the first time you will be eating man's proper food . . . the finest vegetables, the finest grains and seeds and the finest fruits and nuts that exist on earth. You will not suffer and you will not be unhappy. In fact, you will probably enjoy yourself more than you ever have in your life because for the first time you will be eating proper food — nature's food — and the benefits will be manifest with each passing day.

I admit that it will take a few days and sometimes a week or two, for your system to adjust but it will soon happen and you will know how good health can be maintained or regained . . . through proper diet.

The medical profession keeps telling you over and over and over again that arthritic sufferers are sitting ducks for quacks but I am telling you that it is the medical practitioners who are the quacks. They are clutching and holding on to millions of sufferers, whom they are treating with harmful, worthless drugs, and they are extracting a tremendous toll in money for this service . . . even while they admit that there is no known cause and no known cure. I tell you how to get well by the simple expedient of eating natural raw food — the best food that you ever ate in your life. So who are the quacks? I think it is obvious.

I would like to quote now from a book called, "There is Help for Arthritis," by LaRue Stone, an arthritis sufferer for 25 years and Lawrence E. Lamb, M.D., a famed medical columnist:

"I want to emphasize this point only to be certain that the vast number of people with rheumatoid arthritis appreciate in their case, as in individuals who are in better health, an adequate diet is important. Patients with rheumatoid arthritis who live by themselves are particularly apt to have poor diets. The presence of rheumatoid arthritis is not an immunity ticket to the problems of inadequate diet.

"On the general subject of diet and arthritis, you might be interested in knowing what the national headquarters for the Arthritis Foundation says. 'The truth about diets and arthritis may surprise you. It is simply this: There is NO special diet for arthritis. No specific food has anything to do with causing it. And no specific diet will cure it.' The Arthritis Foundation word on diet continues, 'A great deal that you hear and see advertised about special food products for arthritis is outright quackery. It is fantastically profitable for the sellers.' "

I cannot see where anything is fantastically profitable about the thousands and thousands of stores and shops that sell a wide variety of raw vegetables, seeds, fruits and nuts. The profit lies in treating the arthritic sufferers as the medical profession treats them . . . by prescribing drugs, giving various treatments including traction, performing surgery and using X-ray and radium treatments, which only do harm and do not help the poor arthritic sufferer, except to lighten his load by emptying his pockets. The medical profession and the pharmaceutical houses are the prime benefactors.

I would like to quote from a book entitled, "Living With

10

Arthritis," by Dr. A. B. Corrigan.

"There is scarcely one foodstuff which hasn't been blamed for rheumatoid arthritis at some time or another. The victim supposedly either hasn't had enough of it or has consumed too much. But no food will give you the disease. And no food will cure it."

We have some figures here regarding arthritis costs as found on a fact sheet put out by the Arthritis Foundation. They tell us that more than two billion dollars are spent annually for medical care for people suffering from arthritis. They also tell us that three and one half billion dollars in wages and homemaker services are lost annually because of arthritis. Then they tell us the terribly sad news that four hundred million dollars yearly are spent on quack devices and twenty million dollars on research.

Well, obviously the medical profession is still getting five times as much as the so-called quacks and at least the quacks don't cripple you or give you other diseases with the drugs, surgery, X-rays and radium treatments that the medical profession administers. So I think giving four hundred million dollars to the quacks is a better deal than two billion dollars to the medics. Outside information clearly indicates that the Arthritis Foundation's estimate of two billion dollars which accrues to the medical profession annually is a gross under-evaluation — it should be three or four times that much; namely, as high as seven to ten billion dollars annually.

The Arthritis Foundation tells us that arthritis crippling can be prevented by proper diagnosis and interested care. Now I label this a deliberate falsehood, because the medical profession has never in its long history been able to cure a case of arthritis or prevent crippling. Instead, their drugs cause crippling and many other side effects.

It has long been my feeling that every doctor who uses the normal routine in the treatment of arthritis violates the Hippocratic Oath that he has taken because one of the first things that Hippocrates taught was, "Primum est nil nocere." Translated, this phrase means "Above all, do no harm."

There is not one medical doctor alive who can say under oath that drugs, surgery, X-rays and radium do no harm.

In this bulletin it also mentions "Young Arthritics in Action." They are described as a group of young arthritics who have joined together for the opportunity to meet socially, share experiences, and work actively against arthritis, through — you guessed it — fund raising for the Arthritis Foundation. Nothing is mentioned about doing anything to help these young people. They just socialize and help raise money so the Foundation will have more to spend.

I will admit that the Arthritis Foundation does keep records of available sources of common self-help aids and sick-room equipment, such as wheel chairs, crutches and raised toilet seats. However, I maintain that instead of this kind of hanky-panky they should be teaching people about a raw food diet and what substances to avoid so that the arthritic condition will disappear.

The Arthritis Foundation quotes from "The Truth about Aspirin for Arthritis":

"Aspirin is often the best single medicine, but it is often misused, misunderstood, misrepresented or downgraded."

The Arthritis Foundation also gives you a list of books on arthritis, which they recommend to their supporters and readers, but you may be sure that neither this book nor any of my other books will be found on that recommended list. However, I suggest that you read some of the literature they recommend if you want to read nonsense of the highest order and some beautiful, slick specially and professionally prepared Madison Avenue pitches for donations to the Arthritis Foundation.

Now what is most important in the whole Arthritis Foundation bulletin is this sentence, "Your assistance in the form of memorial gifts, donation, or bequest remembrances

12

will help further these programs and overcome arthritis through research."

My suggestion is that all your donations will do is perpetuate the Arthritis Foundation in its business and prevent the arthritics from gaining true knowledge and finding relief from pain and suffering.

At the end of all this on the leaflet they say, "Sending you this literature is made possible by public contributions." So you see, what I say is true.

My bibliography indicates the number of volumes, papers and articles that I have studied to gain information on arthritis and, after reading all this, I suggest that the medical profession is floundering like a fish out of water in the treatment and handling of arthritic conditions. They don't know where to start because by their own admission, they don't know the cause and they don't know the cure. It could be that the quacks don't know the cause or the cure either, but at least they don't prescribe deadly drugs.

I state categorically, without fear of contradiction, that in every single case where they treat an arthritic patient they are contributing harm to the body and definitely contributing to permanent crippling. If any person wishes to investigate part or all of my bibliography to prove the statement that I just made, these documents are available. No normal individual who can read will fail to see the truth of my statements if he takes the time to investigate.

My big beef about the medical profession's treatment of arthritis is that with rare exceptions they still keep on prescribing their harmful methods when they know full well that they do no good and often do much harm.

Not only are some of the doctors' and specialists' words ridiculous but they are often asinine and stupid. If they were to read their own words, which I doubt they have ever bothered to do, I am sure they would be ashamed and embarrassed to think that they would write and print such drivel.

Then they have the audacity to point a finger at quacks who, they claim, take 400 million dollars from the American people. Well, that's surely a case of the pot calling the kettle black.

I openly suggest that arthritis is probably the most profitable disease in America. A patient who is afflicted with this disease must make regular visits to his physician for the rest of his life to receive examinations, prescribed drugs and various other treatments, including surgery. Therefore, it is not too hard to understand why the medical profession and the Arthritis Foundation keep repeating this same old hackneyed story, "There is no cure and there is no known cause." Also, keep in mind that the disease is usually progressive yet no one dies of arthritis . . . they just keep on getting medical treatment.

Incidentally, I might also mention that if a cure for arthritis were found or if the people followed the advice that I give, the medical men would lose their most faithful and best paying clients and the Arthritis Foundation would starve to death . . . which would be a good thing, in my opinion.

Here is what the medical profession offers you in the form of treatment: medication program, drug program, rest program, exercise program, posture rules, splints, walking aids, heat, surgery, prosthetics and rehabilitation.

The medical profession and the Arthritis Foundation, of course, work hand in glove, to tell us about aspirin:

"By all odds, aspirin is the best single drug for most people with rheumatoid arthritis, and the one most frequently prescribed. Because it is such a common household remedy, many people find it hard to believe that it can be 'special' for arthritis.

"It *is special,* because it reduces inflammation in addition to reducing pain . . . and because it is one of the safest drugs available.

14

"But to get its full anti-inflammation effect it must be taken in large doses regularly day after day, even during periods when pain and swelling have subsided and the patient is feeling better.

"Because people vary in their tolerance for aspirin, it should be taken for arthritis only as prescribed by and under the supervision of a physician. For persons who can't take plain aspirin in high dosage, there are other aspirin-type tablets which the doctor can recommend. And for the very few who can't tolerate aspirin at all, the physician can prescribe different medication which is effective."

Imagine paying your physician thousands of dollars, over a period of a lifetime, just to prescribe the 'right' or 'perfect' dose of aspirin! If aspirin is as harmless as they state, with conviction, why must they worry whether the patient takes 3 a day or 23 a day?

If the aspirin manufacturers are not contributing to the general coffers of the American Medical Association and the Arthritis Foundation, it is my feeling that they surely should be. However, they can contribute plenty in many ways besides direct contributions; for example, by advertising and advising the sufferers to consult their physicians.

Nowhere here do they breathe a word to suggest that aspirin creates a whole world of new diseases, including intestinal bleeding, ulcers and possibly cancer.

They go on to tell us about the gold salts and cortisone treatments:

"**GOLD SALTS,** used for years in treating rheumatoid arthritis, reduce the severity of rheumatoid inflammation and are still commonly administered. They are toxic and must be given in very carefully regulated doses. Undesirable side effects must be watched for also with phenylbutazone and antimalarial drugs which are widely used. Indomethacin, a newer anti-inflammatory drug, has relatively minor side effects but is perhaps more useful in other rheumatic diseases,

15

especially osteoarthritis of the hip.

"**CORTISONE** and related steroid drugs are a special problem. They can bring about sensational reduction of pain and inflammation in a matter of hours. The disabled patient suddenly becomes able-bodied again. But steroids have been found to have serious side effects, sometimes worse than the rheumatoid disease. And steroids do not stop the disease process. They merely hide the fact that joint damage is still going on. So although they are still very useful in special situations, they are being prescribed less and less often by arthritis specialists today in the routine treatment of rheumatoid arthritis."

Besides the admitted side effects it has been definitely established that cortisone does contribute to and cause many other diseases. One definitely known is cataract and another is cancer.

There is a cozy working arrangement between the medical profession and the Arthritis Foundation, which sounds like a mutual admiration society. The medical men advise you to consult the Arthritis Foundation and the Arthritis Foundation advises you to see your doctor.

CHAPTER 3

EVERYBODY'S DISEASE

Arthritis has often been called "Everybody's Disease." Statistics tell us that in America more people suffer from arthritis than from any other disease. This gives arthritis a rather unusual and fearful distinction. In fact, it is claimed that only three people out of one hundred will be lucky enough to escape the symptoms and the agony of arthritis by the time they reach the age of 60.

Then we have the experts who add to the above facts, "If you live long enough you will become afflicted with arthritis." However, this has no specific distinction because I have heard the same thing said about cancer ... that is, if you live long enough you will have cancer. If you delve into the matter you will see that degenerative arthritis, properly known as osteoarthritis, is not a disease of old age.

The medical profession claims that the wear and tear of the joints is the cause or contributor to osteoarthritis and yet they tell us that this condition can begin as early in life as twenty.

The researchers and physicians tell us in their literature about arthritis that by the time a person reaches the age of 40 the cartilage at the end of the bones of the affected joints becomes rounded off. They also tell us that this process of wear and tear continues at different rates in different people.

It is maintained by authorities that this "wear and tear" form of arthritis is one of the oldest, if not the oldest, of mankind's ailments and it is found in practically all people and tribes throughout the world.

Now as far as the wear and tear of the bones and joints in the human body is concerned, it is my opinion that this wear and tear can only take place when the body isn't properly nourished and the cells are not being properly regenerated because of a lack of suitable nutrients. All parts of the body are continually being regenerated by the cellular regeneration process and if you fail to supply the body with the essential nutrients which raw food will provide, then this regenerative process is hampered and you can get these cartilage, joint and bone problems. Then, and then only, will they show signs of wear and tear. Then, and then only, can you get arthritis in any of its many forms.

No, my friends, it is not the wear and tear that causes arthritis . . . it is due to an improper diet of mainly cooked, prepared and refined foods that do not regenerate the cells.

On top of that, we read what I consider to be the most alarming and most unusual part of the whole story of arthritis and that is that the skeletons of almost every known species of animal that has ever walked on this earth, including dinosaurs, show clear evidence of arthritis.

When these experts and scientists tell me that the skeletons of almost every known species of animal that has walked on the earth show evidence of arthritis, I call a halt. I cannot accept this. Of course, this is not the first time that I have differed in opinion with the august scientists, investigators, researchers and authorities.

It is my belief that the only animals that definitely show signs of arthritis are domesticated animals that have been fed food provided by man. This would include cats, dogs, cattle, sheep and all other herded or controlled animals.

According to medical literature these are the kinds of

arthritis and I am listing them here so that you can refer to them should the need arise. It will also give you an idea of the various forms and ways that the course of arthritis follows.

There are no doubt many other names given to forms of arthritis but these listed here are generally believed to be authoritative and come from a most respected and reliable medical volume.

Arthritis; Related Disorders

Classification:

"Satisfactory classification of the arthritides and related disorders will not be possible until the causes of several kinds of rheumatic diseases are known. However, the following ha gained fairly general acceptance:

1. Arthritis due to **infection**; e.g., gonococcal, tuberculosis, pneumococcal
2. Arthritis due to **rheumatic fever**
3. **Rheumatoid** arthritis (a) of multiple joints (atrophic arthritis, proliferative arthritis, Still's disease, chronic infectious arthritis)
   (b) of the spine; i.e., rheumatoid spondylitis (Marie-Strumpell arthritis, ankylosing spondylitis, von Bechterew spondylitis, spondylitis ankylopoietica, spondylitis rhizomelica)
4. Arthritis due to direct **trauma**
5. **Neurogenic** arthropathy (Charcot's joint); e.g., tabes dorsalis, syringomyelia
6. **Degenerative** joint disease (osteoarthritis, hypertrophic arthritis, senescent arthritis)
7. **Gouty** arthritis: acute or chronic
8. **Neoplasms** of joints; e.g., synovioma
9. **Hydrarthrosis**, intermittent; e.g., of the knee
10. **Fibromyositis**
11. **Myositis; bursitis**

"Among the many other conditions which may give rise

to pain in or around joints (arthritis or arthralgia) are acromegaly, cyst of meniscus of knee, dermatomyositis, systemic lupus erythematosus, drug intoxication, erythema multiforme exudativum, erythema nodosum, granuloma inguinale, hemophilia, hysteria, leukemia, ochronosis, osteochondritis dissecans, osteochondromatosis, polyarteritis, psoriasis, pulmonary osteoarthropathy, purpura, Raynaud's disease, reflex dystrophy, Reiter's syndrome, scleroderma, septicemia, serum sickness, neuritis and neuralgia."

They do not mention backache, sciatica, lumbago or disc troubles, which I would definitely link in with the others as a form of or an indication of arthritis.

I think arthritis is a mixed-up, rather indefinite term and I suggest that most of the aches and pains in our upper and lower back, in our legs and hips and in our shoulders, arms, hands, wrists and fingers are basically forms of arthritis as recognized or known to the medical or other healing professions.

According to the Arthritis Foundation's booklet, in 1970 there were 17,000,000 with arthritis severe enough to require medical care and each year arthritis claims 250,000 new victims. The figures reveal that there are 5,000,000 with rheumatoid arthritis alone.

I have checked back as best I could and here is the progress of arthritis since the 1940's. In Arnold DeVries's book, "Fountain of Youth," he mentions that in 1940 there were then 6,000,000 people suffering from arthritis. Max Warmbrand in his book tells us that in the 1950's there were 7,000,000 arthritic sufferers. Dr. Paavo Airola in his book, mentioning 1960, tells us that there were 13,000,000 afflicted with arthritis. Then an article written by Dr. John J. Bonica tells us that in 1974 there were 19,000,000 arthritic sufferers. Presumably, these figures refer to the number being treated by the medical profession.

If what the Arthritis Foundation says is true, then there

are many more cases of arthritis in America than we are led to believe because on page 18 of their booklet they say, "Many people with arthritis don't go to a doctor at all."

There are probably 5,000,000 more who seek help from the non-medical healers, such as chiropractors, osteopaths, naturopaths, herbalists and others. Further, we must not ignore the millions who seek help through non-prescription drugs — that is, over-the counter drugs — plus those who seek a cure through spas and various health resorts and institutions. No doubt there are also some millions afflicted where the condition has not developed far enough to be treated and who bear their suffering in silence.

In reading the literature from the Arthritis Foundation, I must admit that I am indeed puzzled because they tell us on repeated occasions that the cause of arthritis is not known and a cure is not known, yet effective treatment methods to control the disease and prevent deformities and crippling are known. In one instance they tell us, "There are likely to be several causes for osteoarthritis rather than one. None is known precisely yet."

I clearly and openly state, with supporting scientific evidence, that the cause of arthritis is known . . . it is a disease caused by refined, fragmented, cooked and chemically treated foods. Arthritis cannot occur or exist in a body that consumes natural foods that are unrefined, uncooked and untreated. No one can show me one single case where arthritis exists in the body of a person who lives on and has always lived on, a diet of natural raw foods. This applies to animals as well as to humans.

Here I present an interesting quotation from the writings of a great author and researcher, Arnold DeVries. It is taken from his book, "The Fountain of Youth":

"Bacteria tend to produce arthritis when the body suffers from a lack of vitamin C. Arthritis can be produced in white rats at will through bacteria injections when the animals' diet lacks vitamin C. But all attempts to give the rats arthritis when their diet is adequate in all respects have failed. Bacteria appear to be a secondary cause of this condition at the most. The real underlying cause is the presence of diseased tissue which has been irritated by toxins. This tissue gives the bacteria an ideal habitat in which they may do their work. To prevent arthritis you must stop doing the things which produce toxemia. You must stop eating devitalized foods which cause a lack of synovial fluid, and you must avoid all intake of inorganic minerals, including common table salt, as some of these have a tendency to cause deposits in the joints."

The experiment proved that arthritis can be caused by a deficiency of Vitamin C, which, incidentally, is found abundantly in raw foods. No one who eats the diet that I suggest could ever be lacking in Vitamin C or, for that matter, in any other vitamin or mineral.

CHAPTER 4

EARLY DETECTION MEANS EARLIER CRIPPLING

It pays to advertise. Business houses throughout America have profitted greatly by sound advertising gimmicks and promotional schemes . . . some ethically questionable but generally equitable and fair.

The medical profession saw this tremendous development in American business and evidently felt that what was good for the business man would also be good for the professional man. So they, too, decided to try to drum up business.

I recall vividly that during the depression years, circa 1930 and even earlier, a doctor was hard-pressed to make a living. I remember doctors sitting in their offices doing nothing, just waiting for someone to get sick and give them a call so they could collect a fee. In fact, doctors in smaller communities were glad to have the local citizenry give them items like eggs, apples and chickens as a means of payment.

Also, during the prohibition days, in some of the Canadian provinces and no doubt in some parts of the United States, doctors were permitted to give prescriptions for liquor where they felt it was needed as a medicine. Most of the doctors that I can recall made a living from making out prescriptions for liquor and most of the prescriptions went to bootleggers. The bootlegger would pay the doctor a fee then go to the government controlled liquor outlet and get a bottle of liquor. The bootlegger would pay for all the prescriptions for liquor that the doctor would give him, so the doctor had a waiting cash customer for every liquor prescription that he was permitted to write.

Well, the medical profession felt that that was not the way they liked things, so they watched the ways and means of advertising used by business firms and institutions to attract business . . . but the medical code prohibits advertising. No doctor can put an ad in the paper and say that he will give you something for a certain fee or the best service you can get would be from him. That is forbidden by the strict ethics of the medical profession.

However, their ethics do not interfere with various societies that are set up throughout America which continually badger the American public to see their doctor, to have themselves examined, to get a check-up and to send a cheque. Nor does it prevent the medical profession from having the pharmaceutical and drug houses hammer away in their advertisments throughout the news and communications media in America, telling people to see their doctor and get their doctor's advice. This barrage of promotion goes on day after day. Yes, more billions are spent on this advertising for doctors than ever anyone would think possible. The advertising expenditures of the drug and pharmaceutical houses border on the fantastic and the benefactor is, in the main, the medical profession.

It is easy to understand why the American Medical Association frowns on spending the practitioner's money on advertising. Why would anyone in the medical profession want to spend his money on advertising when someone else will do it for him? The disease funds and foundations collect millions and spend at least a small amount of it on advertising. The supposed charitable non-profit organizations also receive millions of dollars of free advertising donated by the publishers, radio stations and other advertising media. This is in addition to what the pharmaceutical houses spend on advertising. Oh, yes, the government and all the government agencies recommend seeing your doctor regularly, too.

However, while all these people suggest you see your doctor, I continually point out that going to see a doctor to cure or help you with a disease that he himself has not got licked is a genuine effort in futility.

I very vividly recall this absolutely true incident concerning a friend of mine who was in the hospital suffering from a heart attack. I had been warning him for at least two years about his eating habits but he would not listen.

One day he called me on the phone and said, "Do you know where I am?"

I said, "No, where are you?"

He answered, "I'm in the Hotel Dieu Hospital because I have had a heart attack."

I bluntly replied, "I told you so! I warned you enough times, so it serves you right!"

He snapped back, "That is not what I called up to tell you. You'll get a bang out of this so be quiet and listen. Dr. Brown, who has been my doctor for a long time, didn't turn up this morning. When I asked the nurse where he was, she gave various excuses and eventually said she didn't know. After pressuring her for some time without results, I found out from another doctor that Dr. Brown had had a heart attack himself."

Then my friend went on to say, "I just thought I would acquaint you with the facts because even I can see the irony in the situation . . . especially since you tried so hard to warn me and I know your estimation of doctors."

Elsewhere in this book I cite the example of a doctor who had arthritis. Again, this is really ironic to me.

Here are medical men treating people and prescribing for people with diseases that they cannot handle themselves and are stuck with probably as often as the average individual.

Nothing could be more ridiculous!

I maintain that early detection means earlier crippling because the doctor does not know what to do about your specific arthritic condition except perhaps prescribe aspirin, which any child knows is a sort of haphazard pain killer. But that is not the worst of it. When you go to the doctor in great pain he will probably prescribe cortisone or any one of the cortisone derivatives which invariably create a much more serious and often a much more painful condition than the original arthritis. It is also a broadly accepted fact that some or most doctors treating arthritic sufferers keep trying new drugs which are highly recommended by the detail men representing the pharmaceutical houses, without knowing what the side effects are. The result is that a large number of their patients find themselves suffering from conditions far worse than arthritis.

So I wonder why there is this great clamor and scream, "See your doctor early to prevent crippling" or "Consult your physician" or "Do not go to quacks, go to a doctor." In my humble opinion, nothing could be more ridiculous.

But then you may ask, "Why do you stress that early detection means earlier crippling?"

I maintain that there is good reason for it. For instance, I have a nephew who is a physician — and a mighty good one. He had a family complaint of back trouble that was handed down to all the family. In any event, my nephew, being a doctor, took his own medicine and had his spine fused. Now he has a fused spine so he can't bend and he still has his back pains occasionally.

Well, I, too, had back troubles which I suffered from for years but I eventually found an easier and more sensible solution and I tell people of this means and method of getting rid of back trouble and cite myself as living proof. Incidentally, I recognize back trouble as being a form of arthritis ... perhaps a variation of the form known as spondylitis.

Now if you have arthritic pains and believe the ballyhoo in the newspapers and over the radio, you will go to your physician. What is the first thing he does? He puts you in the hospital for 101 different tests. Unfortunately, the tests, injections, X-rays and other hocus-pocus do kick back . . . but they don't kick back too quickly. Your doctor knows this very, very well and thus he is safe from a lawsuit for malpractice.

It takes weeks, months and often many years for these drugs, treatments, injections and examinations to take their toll . . . and by that time the doctor is home free. This is one of the reasons why in so many instances people are sick, ailing and suffering but the medics cannot find the cause. Yet, the medics themselves and the drugs they prescribe are to blame. This situation has become as common as breathing. More important, hundreds and even thousands of doctors fully realize this but they are helpless unless they use natural methods and run the serious risk of losing their licence and means of a good livelihood.

I suggest that every one of these tests costs you something besides money. That is, it costs you your health in one form or another. They just cannot jab you with needles, extract blood, take X-rays, perform biopsies and do exploratory operations, as well as all the other newfangled tests and experiments on the human body, without doing some harm. So all of this work that they do on your body is a contributing factor to sickness and disease. This is one of the reasons why early detection means earlier crippling.

Yet it is virtually impossible to trace the test, shot, injection, antiobotic or other drug that caused or contributed to the ultimate crippling. I stress that the more treatments of all varieties and kinds that you receive, the greater the risk of permanent crippling.

Then we must not forget that in many cases, if you are

27

in serious pain, they will suggest surgery. Of course, I always remind people that surgery is forever. Once they remove a hip joint or some other part of your anatomy, it is gone forever and if the surgery and replacement parts do not work out properly, you really and truly can be crippled beyond hope.

There is no doubt that many advanced cases of crippling due to worn out hip joints and other bones have been helped through good surgery and prosthetic replacement parts. However, remember that these are foreign objects in the body and could cause trouble or complications at any moment.

I admit that the medical profession does everything humanly possible to try to make you more comfortable, even to the extent of prescribing and fitting you with various gadgets to help ease your pain and suffering. Of course, in the long run, these attempts at medical engineering only cripple you more.

Some of the self-help devices that the medical profession has created or engineered are the following: long handled reachers, such as shoe horns or gadgets that will pick things up for you, built up fork and spoon handles, built up pencils, gadgets that will help you do up buttons, cloth mitts with soap pockets, large handled tooth brushes, raised toilet seats, tap turners to lessen the strain on the fingers, long handled sponges for bathing, sling towels, bath seats, long handled safety razors, magnetic long handled reachers, tilting tea pot stands, tea wagons, bottle cap removers, screw cap removers and hot water holders.

There are various types of crutches, including platform crutches, loft stand crutches, rounded angle grip canes, quad canes, wheel chairs, self lift chairs, and also collapsible steps.

It is undeniable that the medical profession does a very good job of coming up with these aids for crippled arthritis sufferers, but I say it is a poor excuse for telling people how they can correct the condition. In my opinion, these are all poor substitutes for health.

I say that you can get rid of arthritis and let the medical profession keep their super-duper medical engineering. I suggest that the best the medical profession and the Arthritis Foundation can do is prepare one for the life of a cripple . . . with the continual taking of drugs until death do them part and, of course, with a bit of surgery thrown in, too. Oh, yes, there will be some X-rays to see if the condition is worsening . . . with the X-rays contributing in varying degrees to the worsening of the condition.

Another calamitous thing about following medical advice is that they prescribe more sleep for the sufferer. I presume their thinking is that the more the patient sleeps the less he will suffer. They advise as much as 10 to 12 or more hours of sleep every night. To me this is very bad advice because sleep in itself is a prime contributor to crippling, loss of movement and body tone, and body stiffness. Research has clearly indicated that the optimum number of hours of sleep is seven and no more than eight hours should ever be indulged in.

If you want gadgets to allow you to live with your arthritis, if you are content to take drugs for the rest of your days, if you want to undergo surgery and X-rays, and if you want to have replacement parts put into your body, as well as the concomitant drugs that go along with them, then by all means consult your doctor and follow his medical advice.

However, if you want to get rid of your arthritis, if you do not want to be crippled and if you want to regain your health, then follow sane, sensible, logical, proven, natural methods that involve no risk, no money and no gimmicks.

Arthritis sufferers throughout America, wake up! Rid yourself of pain and prevent the crippling of your own body!

CHAPTER 5

MAIN CAUSES OF ARTHRITIS

I claim that arthritis is a disease caused mainly by cooked and processed food. This includes such things as pasteurized dairy products, all of which have been heat-treated because you cannot pasteurize without heat; lack of enzymes due to the fact that all enzymes are destroyed at temperatures above 140 degrees; bread, pies, cakes, cookies, rolls, buns, pizza and any bakery or other product in which wheat is used; a deficiency of various vitamins, specifically the B Vitamins, and E, C and D; and that cup of tea, coffee or other hot beverage.

Many authorities claim that arthritis is caused by metabolic disturbances and an accumulation of toxic substances in the joints. The famed Paul Kouchakoff, M.D., proved conclusively in his experiment (*See page 189*) that all cooked foods are toxic and that some cooked foods are more toxic than others.

"Arthritis is caused by a derangement of the assimilative and eliminative processes of the body."

Please pay attention to this.

Lack of exercise is also a great contributor to arthritis and, of course, as a person becomes afflicted with the disease, he moves about and exercises less and less and this means the condition worsens continually until complete crippling occurs.

It is claimed by a well known authority that the crippling due to lack of exercise comes about because the body normally makes its own cortisone, which is a curing or preventive factor in arthritis, but without exercise the body does not make enough cortisone and thus the crippling occurs. Injections of the cortisone drug are not the answer because it has been proven to cause many more serious conditions than the arthritis itself.

There is no doubt that emotional problems contribute to arthritis but it has been indicated that faulty nutrition is a key factor in emotional disturbances.

A healthy body does not experience aches, pains, discomforts or agony. Nor do the joints in a healthy body become stiff or rigid. When you begin to experience pains or have difficulty in bending that is the time to begin to pay attention. Don't wait until the condition worsens and hope that it will go away on its own.

Recognize the signs early and act. Don't ignore them because the pains are only slight because almost invariably they become worse and worse as time progresses. Act quickly and you can prevent arthritis and be well and have no stiffness or pain or suffering.

As I said, a healthy body does not suffer from backache, lumbago, sciatica, slipped disc, pains in the fingers or the knees or in the back or legs or arms. All of these conditions and signs are clear indications that trouble is brewing. Then the deformities begin to set in and you have difficulty in moving. Learn to recognize the signs of numbness, stiffness, cracking of joints and twinges.

It is unfortunate that the individual usually goes to the doctor when he encounters these conditions. The doctor attempts to allay his fears and most likely prescribes any one of a thousand drugs to make him feel better. However, he does nothing whatsoever to correct the condition.

My investigations and my studies reveal that those

people who tend to use drugs or pills are generally more prone to arthritis than those who abstain from this practice. Just how this contributes to arthritis I do not know at the present moment but it does appear clear that arthritis afflicts those who use pills and drugs to a much greater extent than those who do not use pills and drugs.

I want to stress most emphatically that there is absolutely no connection between advancing years and arthritis. Often a doctor will say, "Well, you are getting on in years, so you can expect to have a few pains."

This is not true. I repeat, there is absolutely no connection between advancing years and arthritis.

I do not advocate the use of oil, be it cod liver oil, safflower oil, sunflower oil, corn oil, soya oil or any other. Don't let anyone mislead you by telling you that your joints must be oiled. All the oil that your body requires is found in raw vegetables, raw grains and raw nuts — in fact, more than the body can possibly use. Yes, the body requires oil, but only natural oil as found in food . . . not the kind in a bottle or can.

No form of sugar should be used — be it white, brown, yellow, raw, molasses, or any other kind.

Now you may say, "But my body needs some form of sugar."

And I say, "You can get all the sugar that your body requires from fresh and dried fruits, as well as vegetables such as carrots, parsnips and others. If you must have some form of sweetening, use good unpasteurized honey — but, I warn, use it judiciously."

Avoid the use of salt in any form and also the use of so-called foods that are known to be salt-carriers. I refer to the various kinds of pickles, sauerkraut, olives and kindred salty products.

I want it clearly understood that I do not recommend or advise the use of any fragmented or refined food — whether it be brewer's yeast, wheat germ, wheat germ oil, cottage cheese, milk powders, condensed, sweetened or skim milk. I maintain that if you want health you must eat only whole foods. If you must use milk, use only raw, unpasteurized milk from a healthy cow.

A poisoned environment, the use of various harmful drugs, faulty nutrition and lack of exercise ... there in a nutshell you have practically all of the basic causes of arthritis.

It must be recognized that heating changes the character of food. The heating of food contributes greatly to arthritis. I contend that boiled water, whether it be used in tea, coffee, postum or any other beverage, is a contributing factor in arthritis. I believe that good, wholesome water from a well, lake or spring contains valuable nutrients but they are rendered unassimilable by the heating.

I cannot understand the logic behind the pasteurization of milk. Any honest nutritionist should know that when you heat a food you reduce or destroy some of its nutritional value. If anyone should doubt the veracity of this statement I suggest that you study the U. S. government's famous publication, Handbook No. 8 of the U. S. Department of Agriculture. Therein you will clearly and unmistakably see that heat does harm food to varying degrees and not only is one element, vitamin or mineral involved, but many. Therefore, there is no question that heat reduces the nutritional value of food.

Pasteurization involves heat and causes destruction of nutrients and, therefore, specifically speaking, changes take place which render many of the nutrients in the milk harmful or unassimilable by the body. Now almost everywhere you are told that milk is a good source of calcium — with which I am in total agreement — but only if the milk is raw, unpasteurized, unheated and untreated. Once the milk has been pasteurized, heated or treated, the calcium can no longer be properly assimilated by the human body. I do not say that the body cannot use the calcium in pasteurized milk but I do say that the body cannot properly utilize the calcium. Yes, the use of pasteurized milk and other dairy products in the American diet is one of the great contributors to arthritis.

If you want information or proof that pasteurization is a factor, I suggest you read the report of Dr. Francis Pottenger's scientifically controlled experiment on cats. The medical profession and the milk industry prefer not to know that this report exists but I suggest you get a copy. Copies are available if you try hard enough.

In my opinion all refined, heated or processed foods are major contributing factors in arthritis.

CHAPTER 6

AN ENZYME DEFICIENCY DISEASE

Gerald Weissmann and his colleagues at the New York University School of Medicine have recognized the fact that many people who are ill are suffering from an enzyme deficiency and they have developed an engineering technique that will take care of this situation.

From Science News, March 29, 1975:

"The enzyme-engineering technique that looks promising, in fact, may also benefit patients with rheumatoid arthritis and gout — two diseases that constitute enzyme leaks rather than enzyme deficiencies.

"In the past, investigators envisioned helping patients with enzyme-based fat and sugar metabolism diseases by giving them enzyme injections. In other words, patients would receive normal versions of those enzymes that they lack. When the investigators attempted to apply the concept, however, they could not sufficiently purify the needed enzymes or get the enzymes to those areas of patients' bodies where they were desperately needed. Finally Roscoe O. Brady and his colleagues at the National Institute of Neurological Diseases and Stroke managed to do so, for two patients with Fabry's disease and for two patients with Gaucher's disease. Both diseases result in excess accumulation of fats due to a faulty fat-metabolism enzyme. The enzyme injections improved the patients' conditions considerably.

"Now Gerald Weissmann of the New York University School of Medicine and his colleagues are taking another tack toward treating patients. Some have Gaucher's disease or Fabry's disease, others have enzyme-based sugar and fat metabolism ailments — Tay-Sachs disease, Niemann-Pick disease, Pompe's disease, the Hunter-Hurler syndrome. Their strategy consists of incorporating normal enzymes, which patients lack, into artificial organelles called liposomes, then injecting the enzyme-laden liposomes into the patients. 'It's generally a way of doing intercellular engineering,' Weissmann explains. . . .

"The New York City rheumatologist anticipates the day where patients with either Tay-Sachs disease or with one of the other 30 or so lysosomal enzyme deficiency diseases will receive liposome-packaged enzymes as regular therapy. 'Patients with these diseases,' as he sees it, 'have a sort of sugar or fat constipation. They get chock-full of these compounds and can't get rid of them. If we can give them normal sugar and fat metabolizing enzymes every couple of weeks, the enzymes should purge them of their abnormal complex sugars or fats.'

"For rheumatoid arthritis and gout patients, enzyme engineering would work somewhat differently, Weissmann anticipates. The reason is that rheumatoid arthritis and gout involve leakage of lysosomal enzymes (causing joint inflammation), rather than defects of lysosomal enzymes.

"Weissmann envisages an elegant rubric. A chemical compound that inhibits lysosomal enzymes would be packaged in liposomes. The liposomes would be incorporated in cells. The cells would be injected in a patient. The liposomes in the injected cells would migrate into the lysosomes of the inflamed cells and release the chemical inhibitor. The inhibitor would stop the lysosomal enzyme leaks. 'Thus nasty lysosomal enzymes,' Weissmann says,

38

'would be inhibited and would no longer cause inflammation.' "

I have gone into detail and given you this information because I wanted to demonstrate to you the maze through which the scientific medical profession goes in trying to correct a simple natural dietary error.

Most of the reactions of metabolism wouldn't occur perceptively in the absence of enzymes at the temperature and in other conditions in which living things exist; and so metabolism is entirely dependent on enzymes.

It is interesting to note that an enzyme is not consumed in its normal process. Therefore, the normal function is continuous in the human system and even when excreted its function continues. If you cook or heat food you kill it but if you eat it raw you enjoy unlimited benefits.

All natural food substances in their normal pristine condition contain their proper quantities of natural enzymes which are put there by nature to fulfill a specific function. They assist in the digestive processes that break down the food and convert it into a form that can be absorbed by the bloodstream to nourish the body and maintain proper cellular regeneration. This has all been provided by nature and all you have to do to get the full benefit of these natural enzymes and remain in good health, is eat foods that contain their full quota of enzymes.

However, the situation as it exists today throughout America and elsewhere is as follows: the vast majority of people eat conventionally. Their diet is made up mostly of cooked, fried, baked, chemically treated and refined, processed food in which all the naturally occurring enzymes have been destroyed. I contend that food thus deprived can never be properly utilized and metabolized by the body, resulting in slowly declining health and various diseases, including arthritis.

Truly, Tobe has been telling arthritis sufferers for almost

20 years that enzymes were the key and the control. Now the medical scientists finally realize there is some truth in this theory . . . but instead of telling their patients to eat raw food — which would be non-remunerative advice — they advise the use of packaged pill-form enzymes or enzyme injections, which no doubt are produced by the big drug corporations.

The doctor will advise the use of these medically engineered enzymes and permit you to follow your bad eating and living habits, which is what most people desire. You will still be able to eat all that crummy, greasy, processed, dead food. However, it would be more fair and more honest if your medical doctor would tell you the truth and allow you to decide which course to follow. But that would not be practising good profitable medicine, would it?

So you have a choice. First, you can follow this medically engineered method and eat the foods that you like and have been taught to enjoy . . . at the same time enjoying poor health with a shortened life span. Second, you can switch over to a raw food diet as John Tobe suggests and eat food containing its full quota of natural enzymes. Then you will enjoy good health and get your full complement of years, without pain or expense, without involvement, without drugs, without treatments and, yes, without doctors.

Here you have the complete picture of the way scientific medicine does it and the way John Tobe advises you to do it.

CHAPTER 7

ESSENTIAL UNSATURATED FATTY ACIDS

Doctor Hugh N. Sinclair of the Department of Nutrition at Oxford University, who is a leading world figure in nutrition, believes that essential unsaturated fatty acids play an important role in the diseases of human beings and animals. He suggests that these EUFA's play an important role in such conditions as arthritis, allergies, bronchial asthma, skin diseases and ulcerative colitis. Furthermore, he suggests that a deficiency of these selfsame acids is a factor in heart disease.

The best source of these EUFA's is edible, viable seeds . . . I repeat, edible, viable seeds. To the best of my knowledge all such seeds contain EUFA's in large quantities: peanuts, soyabeans, coconuts, wheat, rye, oats, flax, sesame, millet, corn, rice, sunflower and cottonseed. They are available in smaller quantities in butter, beef fat, lard, mutton fat, liver fat and milk.

It is important to recognize the fact that while these EUFA's play a vitally important role in human and animal nutrition, it must be remembered that they become rancid and lose much or most of their nutritional value soon after the seed is broken and the oil becomes exposed to the air. So the best way to get your EUFA's or Vitamin F, as Bicknell and Prescott refer to them, is through the ingestion of whole viable seeds.

For your own vital benefit, I suggest .that you study and memorize this most important scientific finding, as quoted by Bicknell and Prescott:

"From the dietetic point of view the most salient property of the unsaturated fatty acids is the ease with which they become rancid, when exposed to the air, through oxidation at their double bonds. The first products of this oxidation are labile peroxides which alter further into keto-hydroxylic derivatives and then either polymerize or undergo disruption with the formation of aldehydic compounds. These products of oxidative rancidity are of the greatest importance since they are not only toxic in themselves causing for instance anemia, but also their presence in food leads to the oxidation and destruction of other substances, so that they may convert diets containing ample carotene and Vitamin A or ample Vitamin E or ample of the Vitamin B Complex into diets deficient in these vitamins."

Thus, the commercial oils used as food not only do not contain assimilable essential unsaturated fatty acids but they convert other good food into harmful or useless substances.

From studying experiments with rats Bicknell and Prescott also noticed, "The symptoms and signs of the fat deficiency disease are retarded and ultimately arrested growth — accompanied by a raised metabolic rate — altered fat and water metabolism, changes in the skin and hair, renal degeneration and impairment of the sexual functions."

To indicate the harm of oxidative rancidity I would like to quote further from Bicknell and Prescott:

"The hydrogenation of the vegetable fats of magarine, while it has the advantage of enabling manufacturers to sell a product which delights shopkeepers by remaining tasteless for many months in a warm room, has, of course, the drawback that much of the essential unsaturated fatty acid is converted to saturated fatty acid."

It is the author's contention that in our modern way of

42

life and method of eating we get little if any of those essential unsaturated fatty acids because today they are milled out in the processing of wheat and other grains. They are not replaced in any way except by some synthetic so-called 'added enrichment' and, therefore, they are not found in our bread, biscuits, cookies, pies or cakes which form a large part of our diet.

Therefore, the bread and bakery products that we eat must be considered an important causative factor in arthritis.

To the best of my knowledge, the role that the unsaturated fatty acids play in arthritis has never been dealt with by any scientist prior to Dr. Sinclair, yet I feel that perhaps the essential unsaturated fatty acids are a very important factor in the causation of arthritis. In fact, they could well be the key to the solution of the puzzle.

CHAPTER 8

VITAMIN D

In the past few years I have done a great deal of reading, researching, inquiring and studying on Vitamin D. This effort was prompted by an inward feeling that Vitamin D is much more important in human health than has so far been recognized by the medical profession, scientists and nutritionists.

It has been established that animals obtain Vitamin D in two ways: First, by devouring animal tissue containing Vitamin D and, second, by the direct action of the sun's rays on the provitamin in or on their own skins. The great researchers, Bicknell and Prescott, state clearly and unmistakably, *"Sunlight acting directly on the body should be the way in which Vitamin D is obtained."*

I quote from Bicknell and Prescott again:

"The action of the sun on the skin is profoundly interesting. The formation of the vitamin appears to occur rather on the skin than in it. Thus birds when they preen themselves remove oil on their beaks from their preen glands and spread it over their feathers, where it is exposed to the sun and activated. It is then either absorbed by the skin or scraped off the feathers by the beak and eaten. The removal of the preen gland makes birds more susceptible to rickets, and prevents ultra-violet light from having any antirachitic effect unless the feet as well as the plumage are irradiated. The fur of animals in a similar way appears to be the place where the vitamin is formed; preventing rats from licking their fur destroys antirachitic effects of irradiation, and owls and young carnivorous birds in captivity have to be given not only the flesh but also the fur of mice or rabbits if they are to thrive. All this suggests that the incessant 'washing' of cats and rabbits and the apparent hunt of monkeys for each other's fleas is really a method of gaining Vitamin D. In man also activation appears to occur on, rather than in, the skin. Helmer and Jansen found that the fat washed off the bodies of athletes who had been exposed to irradiation before taking violent exercise was antirachitic, while fat from the skin of the athletes who had not been irradiated had only a trivial potency. Irradiation of this fat made it potent. Further, the ultra-violet rays of the sun penetrate only some 0.1 mm. to 1.2 mm. through the skin, so that activation must occur at least close to the surface. Possibly the old belief that too much washing makes babies fretful is due to the removal of their Vitamin D leading to the fretfulness of rickets. After sunbathing it appears possible that swimming is a mistake, the activated fat being washed off the skin before it has had time to be absorbed."

It is claimed by some of the best authorities that food as a source of Vitamin D is generally not important in human nutrition. Studies reveal that of all creatures on the face of the earth only man and, at that, only man living in temperate and cold climates is driven to use food as an alternative to the sun and atmosphere as a source of supply of Vitamin D.

While Vitamin D is poorly represented in food it is found in dairy products, egg yolk, fish-liver oils, some fish, liver, oysters and yeast . . . but it is my serious contention that of this list only the oysters, liver and fish are natural foods for man. Thus, foods containing Vitamin D appear to be rather scarce. I do not believe that man was intended to obtain his nourishment from milk and, therefore, I do not believe that you were ever intended to get Vitamin D in this manner.

Unfortunately, green vegetables do not contain Vitamin D in any appreciable quantities. Of all the natural vegetable foods, only mushrooms have clearly demonstrable quantities of Vitamin D.

I would bring to your attention the fact that Vitamin D is found in seeds and grains — that is, in the germ or the living component of the seeds. Remember this fact — it is important!

There is a generally mistaken impression concerning the source of Vitamin D from the atmosphere and that is that Vitamin D comes directly from the sun's rays. In other words, it is generally believed that your body cannot absorb or acquire Vitamin D unless the sun is shining. Now this has been scientifically proven to be erroneous. The body can readily absorb all the Vitamin D it requires from the atmosphere even if the sun is not shining or if it has not shone for days. The body's absorption of Vitamin D takes place from the action on the skin by the atmosphere . . . but only if you haven't interfered with the natural coating of oil that the body has on its skin.

It has been established that Vitamin D is absolutely essential for the metabolism of calcium and phosphorus and is essential for normal development of bones and teeth and for their continued maintenance. So it is important that nothing be done to impair the body's ability to absorb natural Vitamin D from the atmosphere.

I want to impress upon you the importance of avoiding the use of soaps, detergents, various cosmetics, hair preparations and oils, perfumes and other beauty accoutrements on man and beast because they will prevent the absorption of Vitamin D. Let me state emphatically that any and all of the cosmetics, detergents, soaps and shampoos that are used are detrimental.

The usual complaint that I hear when I tell people not to use soap for bathing is, "How will I get my body clean?"

My reply is, "Water and a good brushing and some rubbing will do far more good for the body than the use of all of those substances mentioned."

I have not used soap in my bathing for almost 20 years, nor do I use any shampoos or other preparations on my head. I do use shaving soap but I assure you, it does cause me some uneasiness. I may have to grow a beard! I must also admit that I do use soap on my hands when I have been doing some chores and my hands have become greasy or stained.

If you insist on using soaps and cosmetics, I understand there is a firm in America that makes strictly organic cosmetic preparations which are claimed not to be harmful but actually beneficial. I certainly would investigate and try these products rather than the products made with harsh chemicals.

It has been my contention for many years that it was never intended that the human body get supplies of Vitamin D from any other source than from the atmosphere. It is my sincere belief, supported by growing amounts of scientific data, that Vitamin D obtained from other sources can actually do harm and be toxic to the human body if ingested in large quantities.

As proof of this statement I would like to quote from an article that appeared in the U. S. News & World Report of August 13, 1973:

"Vitamin D — turns calcium and phosphorus in foods into bone. Lack of it in children causes rickets; in adults, porous, brittle bones. Natural sources: eggs, butter, fish-liver oils. Overdose dangers: can cause serious blockages in soft tissues of the liver and kidneys, sometimes leading to death."

So I feel that I must warn against the use of a Vitamin D supplement. There have been countless incidents where overdoses of Vitamin D have caused serious consequences.

This may surprise you but it is a scientific fact that doctors prescribe doses of Vitamin D ranging from 50,000 to 600,000 International Units. I think there is little or no danger of getting an excess of Vitamin D from the atmosphere and, therefore, I recommend that this is where the body should obtain it.

It is of great interest to note that human milk contains only small quantities of Vitamin D . . . yes, even as little as 40 I.U.'s per quart of human milk. This would also indicate that nature did not intend human beings to get their Vitamin D from milk.

In the next chapter I will attempt to explain the various ways in which Vitamin D is linked with the metabolism of many minerals and elements which occur naturally in food.

CHAPTER 9

METABOLISM OF CALCIUM AND PHOSPHORUS

This chapter is one of the most important chapters, if not the most important chapter in this volume. So read and heed!

Vitamin D is known as the antirachitic or the calcifying vitamin and it is claimed that the early history of Vitamin D is the history of rickets. It is a depressing history: a history of perfect clinical observation on the cure of the disease being forgotten again and again for more than a century and a half.

Rickets first became recognized as a definite disease by the medical profession in the last half of the seventeenth century. The name rickets, according to Skeat, is an old English word: the adjective rachitic was forced into our language by the mistaken desire of lovers of the classics to give rickets a Greek derivation.

According to my medical dictionary, under rickets: "A form of osteomalacia in children. It results from deficient deposition of lime salts in developing cartilage and newly formed bone, causing abnormalities in shape and structure of the bones."

Under osteomalacia, we read, "Softening of the bones. A disease marked by increasing softness of the bones, so that they become flexible and brittle, thus causing deformities. Occurs in adults and chiefly in women.

51

"Symptoms: Rheumatic pains in the limbs, spine, thorax, and especially the pelvis; anemia and signs of deficiency disease; progressive weakness. Finally death occurs from exhaustion."

Again I would like to quote something by Bicknell and Prescott that I think is of keen interest:

"The eighteenth century added little to the history of rickets until toward its end when cod liver oil was first used in medicine, though apparently in Scotland and Northern Europe cod liver oil had been popular for many years with the peasants as a cure for rickets and other diseases.

"In 1782 Dr. Robert Darley wrote to Dr. Thomas Percival an account of his use of cod liver oil, which was so highly successful that the poor clamoured for it, though its smell and taste were loathsome as it was made by 'heaping together the livers of the fish, from which, by gentle putrefaction the oil flows very beautifully.' Percival recommended peppermint to conceal the taste — advice which a century and a half of further experience has not bettered. But it must be admitted that the earliest account of the value of cod liver oil did not stress its value in rickets: in fact, only two children were reported, the other cases being arthritis or rheumatism."

The reason I make the analogy between rickets and arthritis is because in both conditions the importance of calcium and phosphorus has been definitely proven. This was established by McCollum and Mellanby. It is claimed with authority that rickets only develops if these two elements are badly balanced in the diet. In experiments with rats that were deficient in Vitamin D, rickets did not occur unless the calcium and phosphorus intake was not balanced.

Here are more excerpts from Bicknell and Prescott:

"The body appears to have no power to regulate the amount of Vitamin D it absorbs in the food; whether it can regulate that formed in the skin by irradiation is unknown.

But as the latter appears to be the natural way of acquiring vitamin D experiments suggesting the value of a high consumption of the vitamin should only be accepted if the results are the same as given by irradiation. Any results which appear to suggest feeding is better than irradiation may mean that they are not truly better, but are the effect of abnormal stimulation. If growth is taken as the criterion for measuring the correct dose of vitamin D we should know what is optimum growth. We do not. . . .

"The effects of vitamin D are best explained, though it must be admitted not completely, by considering that its action is primarily on phosphorus metabolism throughout the whole body. Thus vitamin D not only mobilizes phosphorus from the tissues, so aiding its combination with calcium by converting organic phosphorus into an inorganic form, but it also has an effect on the metabolism of phosphorus during muscular work."

For many years I have been pointing out the questionability of the value of food supplements in the diet. I say that if you want calcium or any other element or mineral in your body, you have to get it via good food where it is accompanied by the other essential elements, vitamins and nutrients. Just adding calcium to your diet, in the form of bone-meal, gelatin, dolomite and other such substances as some nutritionists suggest, is wrong because the proper balance with phosphorus and other elements is not maintained. Therefore, it can cause harm instead of benefit to the body.

The following information comes from an article entitled "Intestinal Absorption of Calcium," by M. R. Wills.

"The rate of absorption of calcium from the intestine depends on a number of factors, including age, body requirements, previous dietary calcium intake, the absolute amount of calcium in the gut, the availability of calcium in the gut and the effects of other substances on the availability of calcium for absorption, bile secretion and fatty acids, parathryroid hormone, and the cholecalciferol. . . .

"Studies of calcium absorption in man suggest that calcium absorption diminishes with age in both sexes, starting at the age of 55-60 years in women and 65-70 years in men. By the ninth decade in both men and women there was a significant degree of malabsorption of calcium. The mechanism for this diminution in intestinal calcium absorption with age is not clearly defined. Bullamore et al. suggested that it may well be due to cholecalciferol deficiency, either from inadequate endogenous synthesis or inadequate dietary intake of exogenous cholecalciferol. . . .

"There is, however, no unequivocal evidence that a habitually low intake of calcium is harmful — indeed there is evidence that low intakes are compatible with normal skeletal homeostasis. In long-term calcium-balance studies in healthy people calcium absorption from the intestine increases as an adaptation to a low-calcium diet. . . .

"The effect of phosphate on the intestinal absorption of calcium, plasma-calcium homeostasis, and bone mineralization is dependent on the dietary calcium intake and on the ratio of calcium to phosphate in the diet. The intestinal mechanisms for the absorption of calcium and phosphate are linked, and although active calcium transport takes place in the absence of phosphate there is evidence that the presence of phosphate in the diet is essential for the optimal absorption of calcium."

From another part of the Willis study we quote:

"Vitamin D is the name given to a group of steroid compounds which possess antirachitic properties; cholecalciferol (vitamin D_3) is the naturally occurring compound in man. Cholecalciferol is formed on the skin from 7-dehydrocholesterol with cleavage of the B-ring carbon-carbon bond between C9 and C10 of the steroid structure. The cleavage is achieved by irradiation with ultraviolet light in the wave-

54

lengths of 280-305 nm. The , endogenous synthesis of cholecalciferol in the skin is related to the degree of skin pigmentation, to the amount of available ultraviolet light in solar and sky radiation, and to the duration of exposure to ultraviolet light."

However, there is another factor involved here which has not as yet been mentioned. Let us assume that we keep the body in such a position and shape that it can absorb Vitamin D from the sun and the atmosphere. This is all within the realms of possiblity. I am talking about a person, young or old, male or female, who does not use cosmetics, harsh soaps, detergents, pharmaceuticals or other substances that would remove the oily covering from the body and otherwise impair or prevent the body from absorbing Vitamin D.

This person is absorbing all the Vitamin D the body requires, yet he is not getting Vitamin D. How does this happen? Very easily — if he uses mineral oil in any manner, shape or form, even as a laxative. This product is widely sold throughout America and widely used because it does make a pleasant, easy-going, effective laxative.

Unfortunately, mineral oil is called by many other names so you may not recognize it as mineral oil. Here I am giving you a list of names by which mineral oil or petrolatum liquid is known: liquid paraffin, mineral oil, white mineral oil, Nujol, kaydol, alboline, paroleine, saxol, adepsine oil, glymol. Mineral oil prevents the absorption of the oil-soluable vitamins, of which Vitamin D is one.

Mineral oil prevents or interferes with the absorption of minerals as well as vitamins and in this case it prevents the absorption of calcium. In other words, you may be getting plenty of Vitamin D and you may be getting plenty of calcium from your food, yet you have arthritis or other diseases because the mineral oil prevents or interferes with the body's absorption of calcium. Another point for your consideration . . . mineral oil is widely used as a vehicle for drugs, especially for drugs applied to the nasal mucosa.

It is my contention, based upon many investigations and studies, that hydrogenated oil acts in a similar manner to mineral oil. In the processing of the oil, by the injection of finely pulverized nickel as a catalyst into the oil to make it hydrogenated, it is turned into a plastic fat. This hydrogenated oil or plastic fat is one of the main components of margarine and I suggest that this oil interferes with the absorption of Vitamin D and minerals like calcium. Thus the body is starved for calcium and, since there is no calcium to combine with the phosphorus which is so badly needed by the body, the body is starved for phosphorus, too.

Another interesting aspect regarding calcium metabolization comes to light in the fact that refined fats and oils have lost their ability to retain and utilize calcium. Therefore, any person who uses any quantity of the various oils on the market today, which are invariably refined fats and oils, will have a calcium metabolization problem.

If you take the trouble to check the statistics, you will find that the number of arthritics began to rise when margarine was approved by the powers that be and began to appear on the open market in America. There is a direct link between the increased quantity of margarine used by the American people and the incidence of arthritis. Check it through the past 30 years and you will find that I speak the truth.

CHAPTER 10

BREAD AND OTHER WHEAT PRODUCTS

We have been taught for centuries that bread is the staff of life, and so it continues even to this day. Well, I maintain that bread, along with all the other wheat products, is one of the foremost contributors to the cause of arthritis.

Would it be wrong to say that bread plays a bigger, more important role in the American diet than any other food? There is no doubt we use more bread than we do sugar, more bread than we do meat and more bread than we do milk.

There are no accurate figures — at least I couldn't locate any — but estimates reveal that the percentage of bread and other wheat products in the American diet runs as high as 60% of the total caloric intake. Now this may be an exaggeration but when I compared this with the amount of bread consumed in our home when I was a child and then later on in my own home in my early married days, I had to accept the shocking conclusion that bread and other wheat products could very easily make up 60% of the caloric intake of the American people.

At a casual glance it seems ridiculous to suggest that wheat products play such an enormous role in our diet. However, if you take into consideration such things as spaghetti, macaroni, ravioli, noodles, bread, cake, pie, cookies, buns, rolls, muffins, crumpets, cream of wheat, wheatlets, crackers, biscuits, bagels, matzos, rusks, pizza and dumplings, I am afraid you would find that wheat products do form 60% of the caloric intake of the American people.

Now it makes little or no difference whether the bread you eat is white, brown, rye, seven grain or black, it is still mainly wheat. Even the best rye bread on the market contains 40% to 70% wheat. Just how much wheat is found in the various packaged cereals like shredded wheat, crispies, crunchies and granola I am not able to say. Then bear in mind that because of its comparatively low price and its high food value, wheat is used by food processors in many other ways . . . in soups, gravies, sauces, chowders and even in candy and chocolate bars. Then too, we bread our fish, chops and various other products for deep-frying.

However, the moment I suggest eliminating or cutting down on the amount of these products containing wheat, I am greeted with howls of displeasure, shock and bewilderment. Invariably people say, "What are we going to eat to replace them?"

Well, the answer is fairly easy. As foods that are as satisfying and nourishing as bread you could use potatoes and other root vegetables, as well as rice and other grains and seeds. On the other hand, these foods do not lend themselves to making sandwiches nor to the smearing on of butter, margarine, jam, jelly, honey or peanut butter, as does bread.

Remember, I was loathe to part with bread. I love the stuff, plain or toasted and especially the mighty good bread that my wife bakes. When I cut down on the bread in my diet, naturally my butter consumption went down drastically, too, and the use of jams and jellies was totally eliminated. The amount of honey and peanut butter also was cut down drastically. To say the least, this all left a tremendous void that was difficult to fill.

Now don't run off with the idea that it will be all right if you get organically grown wheat, grind it yourself and

58

make your own bread. It won't! I know because I have tried them all . . . not once, not twice, but over and over again. Personally, I avoid bread in any form and have done so for many years. However, I still have it placed before me whenever I go out, but in the main I resist. I must confess that I still occasionally indulge in a slice or two of good bread.

There are eminent authorities who claim that it is the lack of roughage in the diet that is a factor in arthritis. I will not dispute this argument but as far as pains in the back, arms, hands, fingers, legs, shoulders, etc. are concerned, it makes little or no difference whether it is genuine, homemade, whole wheat bread that is loaded with fibre or the puffy, fluffy, bleached, impoverished and enriched white bread from the supermarket. They are all bread and they all bring devastation to me every time I eat them. The only difference is that those who eat refined bread have their back pain with constipation, while I have my back pain without constipation.

There is not the slightest doubt in my mind that the refined white bread would contribute to an arthritic condition sooner and more virulently than the whole wheat bread from flour you grind yourself. This is simply due to the fact that you can eat much more of the puffy, refined white bread than you can of the coarser whole grain bread.

Remember, too, when you eat the normal white bread that is offered everywhere, you are being cheated out of the essential nutrients found in whole wheat. It is claimed that refining removes from wheat a significant amount of protein — about 11%. From documented figures I read that in the process of milling white flour, most of eight natural and essential vitamins are removed from the wheat and three chemical, synthetic ones are added to enrich the flour. In other words, you lose eight whole, complete vitamins in the process and then the millers add three synthetic ones and they call this enrichment. Personally, I doubt whether the body can assimilate the synthetic substances.

Henry A. Schroeder, M.D., a world authority on trace minerals points out in his important new book, "Trace Elements and Man":

"The milling of wheat into refined white flour removes 40% of the chromium, 86% of the manganese, 76% of the iron, 89% of the cobalt, 68% of the copper, 78% of the zinc and 48% of the molybdenum, all trace elements essential for life or health. Only iron, and that in a form poorly absorbed, is later added to flour. The residue, or millfeeds, rich in trace elements, is fed to our domestic animals. And by the same process, most of eight vitamins are removed from wheat, three are added to make the flour enriched; millfeeds are rich in vitamins. Similar depletion of vitamins and essential trace elements occurs when rice is polished and corn meal refined. Likewise, most of the bulk elements are removed from wheat: 60% of the calcium, 71% of the phosphorus, 85% of the magnesium, 77% of the potassium, 78% of the sodium, which appear in the millfeeds."

Now there is no doubt that the elimination of these important food components from the white bread could be a vital link in the causation of arthritis.

Dr. T. L. Cleave, M.R.C.P. (Lond.) Surgeon-Captain Royal Navy (Retd.) proved that degenerative diseases, of which arthritis is by far the most prevalent, are caused by concentrated foods, especially white flour and sugar, which have had the fibre refined out of them.

It has been stated that in the United States more than 28,000,000 people a year go to their medical doctor because they have trouble with their backs and then, through the various forms of treatment, including surgery, their backs are manipulated and massaged, twisted and jerked, stretched and straightened, heated and sprayed, and they are given injections and drugs.

Now I claim that at least an equal number, or maybe more, go to a chiropractor or to a masseur or to other types of practitioners who treat their back troubles in various ways . . . from diet to neck and limb twisting and other manipulative procedures. This would mean that close to 60,000,000 people every year go through these maneuvers because of back troubles that occur and disappear and then reoccur. These back troubles are usually categorized as being a form of arthritis. Of course, I did not mention discs which are part of the back syndrome.

Whether you accept it or choose to ignore my serious findings, I claim that most of those 60 million sufferers could ease or totally rid themselves of this painful problem by following my simple, straightforward counsel.

Well, I have proven to myself, to my wife and to many of my friends, readers and associates that most of the pains and aches in one's shoulders, hands, legs and back can be eliminated by giving up bread or wheat in any form. Most people ridicule the idea and would not dream of trying it even though they may suffer with one or many pains. Those who do try it and stick to it achieve success almost without fail.

Unbelievable, but true! And you can prove it to yourself in very quick order. Just stop eating bread or wheat in any form for as little as three to five days and you will notice a difference.

CHAPTER 11

TEA FOR TWO

I doubt if any other researcher has ever considered the fact that the beverages we drink could be a causative factor in arthritis. Well, I don't know why but somehow, even as a younger man, I always associated little old ladies sipping tea with arthritis.

Human beings are really not very clever or they would not keep repeating the same mistakes made by their fathers, their grandfathers and their great-grandfathers. Perhaps I am wrong but it is my opinion that man does not learn but just follows along in his predecessors' footsteps . . . making the same mistakes they did.

We all love our cup of tea or coffee or it could be postum or even a herb tea and through the centuries a cup of tea or coffee has been recognized as a sign of conviviality. Of course, nowadays they have switched over to beer, wine, liquor and other alcoholic beverages. However, basically, a cup of tea was a specific sign of sociability. Whenever one met a friend or associate it was always, "Let's have a cup of tea."

Do you recall, probably even in your youth, seeing the incrustation that lined the inside of a teakettle that had long been used in the household? By banging it or tapping it sharply with a solid instrument, you could chip some of it off. When you held the chip in your hand, you could see that it was like a piece of stone or rock. What it really was, of course, was lime. This incrustation of lime had gradually built up until it became quite thick after many hundreds or thousands of cups of water had been boiled in the kettle.

This indicates that water contains things other than hydrogen and oxygen. In fact, you would be really astounded if you investigated and found out just what water does contain. No, I am not talking about polluted water, dirty water, muddy water or water unfit for human consumption. I am talking about what we know as good, potable water — be it from a well, from a spring, from a stream or from a lake.

I have watched birds, cattle, horses, dogs, cats and most animals native to our land and I have noticed that they prefer surface water to fresh water from a stream, lake or spring. I maintain that they seek it out in preference to other water because the surface water contains more of these active minerals and substances that I mentioned. You have no doubt made this observation, too.

For centuries it has been generally accepted by the scientific fraternity that water contains inorganic minerals which the body cannot assimilate. However, studies reveal to me that water contains many important organic minerals and other substances which are assimilable and are necessary for good health. I have battled this out on many occasions with many so-called authorities and laymen, but they always argue that the elements, the minerals and any other substances in the water cannot be absorbed and utilized by the body.

If you are interested in documentation, Dr. W. D. Keller of the University of Missouri, who did major work on glacial streams and waters, proved without a shadow of doubt that water does contain vitally important nutrients and furthermore that these nutrients can be absorbed and utilized by the human body. This work was entitled, "Glacial Milks and Their Laboratory-Simulated Counterparts", by W. D. Keller, University of Missouri, Columbia, Missouri and A. L.

Reesman, Department of Geology, University of North Dakota, Grand Forks, North Dakota.

"But how does all this affect the arthritis sufferer?" you may be wondering.

Well, when you drink cool or cold water in its natural form, the body can utilize the nutrients found in water. However, when you cook, boil or heat water, the body cannot properly utilize these very valuable minerals or nutrients. Therefore, they are malabsorbed and find their way into places in the body where they do not belong and thus we have contributing factors in bursitis, spurs, spondylitis and a dozen and one other forms of arthritis, as well as other diseases.

At this time I would like to again bring to your attention those little things called enzymes. Enzymes are found in all natural substances, but enzymes are heat labile and are destroyed when they are heated to 140 degrees Fahrenheit or more. Thus, the key to the lock is lost and the body cannot properly metabolize the substances found in water that has been boiled.

I am suggesting that boiled water, whether used in making tea, coffee or some other beverage, is a positive contributor to arthritis and probably a much greater contributor than is generally known.

If you want to get rid of this contributor to arthritis, do not seek any substitutes. Just drink plain, ordinary, untreated and unheated water, preferably fresh from a well or a spring. Do not look for substitutes . . . there are none! You will just have to forgo the delight and pleasure of drinking hot beverages . . . but, then, what's wrong with sipping a nice cool glassful of good potable water?

Yes, the more I examine the situation, the more convinced I am that all of our boiled beverages are harmful to some degree.

CHAPTER 12

FROZEN FOODS AND VITAMIN K

Although I do not have much proof at the moment, I believe that frozen foods are a contributing factor in arthritis.

The fact that freezing destroys Vitamin K is important in itself because, after all, Vitamin K is a vital substance in the diet of human beings. Just how important, scientists have yet to discover but they do know that Vitamin K is essential for normal blood coagulation. In fact, it is called Vitamin K for Koagulation which is the Danish spelling of our word 'coagulation'.

The specific purpose of Vitamin K in the body is for the formation of prothrombin and thus it is known as the antihemorrhagic factor. Its deficiency prolongs blood clotting time and causes hemorrhages. Vitamin K is widely used in surgical practices because it helps to eliminate prolonged bleeding in operations and in biliary tract of jaundiced patients.

Bicknell and Prescott tell us that, according to A. J. Quick, prothrombin is composed of calcium and two separable components, one of which is stable and appears to be related to the oxidation-reduction systems of the blood, the other being heat labile and inactivated by dicumarol. Heat labile means it is harmed or destroyed by heat.

Vitamin K occurs in greates abundance in all green leafy

vegetables . . . spinach, kale, cabbage, cauliflower and alfalfa being especially rich sources. It is also found in green peas, carrot tops, blackstrap molasses, liver, egg yolk, oats, wheat, rye, soybean oil and fish liver oil. You will note that Vitamin K is found most abundantly in green leaves.

It is also interesting to note that Vitamin K is synthesized from coal tar and such Vitamin K is supposed to be four times as potent as the natural Vitamin K.

To the best of my knowledge no scientist has done any testing to indicate the value of Vitamin K to arthritis sufferers but they keep referring to the tremendous amount of Vitamin K units found in cabbage, cauliflower petals, alfalfa, pine needles, etc.

Back in 1935, two researchers — Almquist and Stokstad — discovered that alfalfa meal is a potent source of Vitamin K and all the data is given in their research paper called "Haemorrhagic Chick Disease of Dietary Origin" and it appeared in the Journal of Biological Chemistry in 1935, p. 111, Vol. 105.

I am suggesting that Vitamin K plays an important role in the prevention and relief of arthritis and foods containing adequate quantities of this vitamin should be included in the diet of every arthritis sufferer and those who wish to avoid arthritis. Since Vitamin K is destroyed by freezing, frozen food may be almost as big a factor as cooked food in the cause of arthritis. I strongly recommend that neither frozen nor cooked foods be used in the diet of anyone suffering from arthritis.

It has been brought to my attention that most vegetables are blanched before they are frozen, which means they are dipped into hot or boiling water. Most of the frozen foods are cooked again before they are eaten. We know Vitamin K is damaged in the freezing and that enzymes are killed in the heat or boiling water treatment. Therefore, frozen food becomes less and less of a food and more and more of a wasted food.

We have practically eliminated all forms of frozen food from our diet and this includes meat, fish, fruits and vegetables. I suggest that you do likewise. Keep frozen foods only for emergency purposes but for health purposes make sure that you get fresh food.

I have frequently been asked for an alternative to freezing when you want to store some food in time of surplus for the time when there will be a need. Well, I suggest drying food. Today there are many good drying units on the market. We dry all our surplus fruits and vegetables. We even dry mushrooms and a neighbor of mine just finished drying venison. He asked me to sample a piece and when I did, all I could say was that it tasted superb.

There you have my answer to the food storage problem — drying — but I must warn against the use of high heat in drying. Make sure the temperature does not get above 140 degrees Fahrenheit.

I would like to bring to your atttention an interesting piece of research work that sheds some light on the importance of Vitamin K in the diet of man.

According to a paper written by researcher W. B. Rawls entitled, 'Vitamin K in other than Haemorrhagic Diseases,' published in the Southern Medical Journal, 1941, 34, 1266, he observed hypoprothrombinaemia in patients suffering from rheumatoid arthritis. This indicates that patients suffering from arthritis should never take aspirin because aspirin actually causes hypoprothrombinaemia. Therefore, it is clear that the use of aspirin is positively contraindicated and could only worsen the arthritic sufferer's condition. If you do use aspirin, then it would be very wise to fortify yourself with extra quantities of Vitamin K.

I want to point out that mineral oil and sulfa drugs will definitely destroy the Vitamin K in your body. There are probably many other drugs that harm and destroy your

Vitamin K as well as those mentioned.

CHAPTER 13

ARTHRITIS AND YOUR EMOTIONS

Many authorities and experts claim that emotion is a factor in arthritis, but I do not accept this belief.

Some of these people link the onset of arthritis with certain traumatic or tragic events such as an accident, a bereavement, a shock, a family quarrel or being fired from a very good job. A report of a thirteen year study at the Cornell University Arthritis Clinic would have us believe that such emotional disturbances as financial problems, long hidden and smoldering resentments, as well as broken homes, can cause arthritis.

It is my feeling that it is not emotion that is a factor in arthritis but the onset of the arthritic condition that builds up one's emotions practically to the breaking point.

Arthritis doesn't spring up overnight but there are various symptoms that slowly appear without the individual realizing what is going on. It is felt in hundreds of different ways ... such as, a slackening in mobility with aches in the arms, legs, wrists, fingers and even in the jaws and teeth; twinges here, a pain there, a crick in the neck, a sensitive elbow or a painful knee.

These indications have been cropping up for days, weeks, months or even years. There hasn't been anything severe enough to make one suspect the onset of arthritis but it has just been tantalizing enough to make one tense, out of sorts or edgy. It is then that our emotions come into play and it is this gradual build-up that eventually triggers emotional stress and strain.

We do know that emotion represents a moving agitation, tumult or excitement within the human, which definitely does affect our mental status. Furthermore, emotion can involve the feelings of affection, pain, desire and, yes, even hope. Well, when all of these factors are weighed and carefully taken into consideration, it is my sincere belief that it is the arthritic condition that brings about the emotions, as I have mentioned, and not the emotions that are the cause of the arthritic condition.

Through the years I have heard of and been involved in predicaments where a traumatic situation brought about the onset of a disease. A case in point was my eldest brother. When he was told by phone that my father had been killed in an accident he suffered a tremendous emotional upset because he was very close to my father. From that day on he became a diabetic. He blamed the shock of this tragic occurrence as being the cause of his diabetes. However, I know full well that he had been living and eating in a manner that would bring on diabetes and there is no doubt in my mind at all that his diabetes was earned. The shock just triggered the diabetes and brought it to the fore.

I am sure that you know of cases, as well as I do, where a man in a very competitive business is suffering a great deal of pain from ulcers. He claims that the stress of business caused the ulcers. The same story holds true for migraine headaches, intestinal disorders and even cancer, which are claimed to be brought on by emotional strain. What they mean to say is that the rat race is to blame. My conclusion after many years of observation, is that they are wrong.

To accept the thesis that emotion or stress can cause arthritis is to accept the fact that it is strictly mind over matter. I do not think you can talk yourself into a disease any more than you can talk yourself out of a disease . . . or perhaps I should have said, think yourself into or out of a disease. By this I do not infer that there is no such thing as psychosomatic disease, because I know there is, but I do not believe emotion and stress can bring on arthritis or any other degenerative disease.

If you eat right, live right and do not repeatedly commit biological offences against the body, you will have a healthy body free of arthritis. But if you violate biological laws as far as eating and living habits are concerned, which is true of 99% of the people in America, then you will have to suffer the consequences, which in many cases is arthritis. By the same rule, if you correct your living habits and remove all harmful and contributing factors, then good health should return . . . and it will!

I am quite willing to concede and accept the fact that pent up emotions and stress, built up by tension, mental disquietude and lack of harmony, can trigger many physical conditions or diseases. However — and this I consider of great importance — it can only bring on these various conditions if the groundwork has already been well laid down by years of improper diet and wrong living habits.

I know many people, as I am sure you do, who sort of emote all over the place at the drop of a hat. That is, they will either cry or laugh at the least provocation. However, they do not necessarily have arthritis, ulcers, diabetes, heart disease, intestinal disorders or cancer. The reason why is clear . . . the groundwork has not been laid down by violations of natural, biological law.

I read somewhere that Professor Hans Selye of Montreal, the renowned and celebrated authority on stress, believes that many diseases including arthritis are caused by stress. Of course, I do not believe that this is true and the proof is Professor Hans Selye himself who has suffered from arthritis

73

for many years. Surely, a man who knows as much about stress and tension as Professor Hans Selye could have prevented or avoided the condition. He has a prosthetic hip and he claims that he is doing very well with it.

The proponents of the stress factor in arthritis point out that Vitamin C is known as the anti-stress vitamin. They claim that Vitamin C stimulates the adrenal glands and increases the production of cortisone. Well, if Vitamin C is the anti-stress vitamin and stress is due to lack of Vitamin C, then the answer is to take lots of Vitamin C and you won't have stress and thus, no arthritis. This to me is a gross over-simplification!

From an experiment recounted in the American Journal of Clinical Nutrition, November, 1962, we learn that emotional upsets increase the retention of calcium. It was discovered that the amount of increase was in exact ratio to the amount of tension experienced. In response to this finding I would mention that the drinking of pasteurized milk also causes retention of calcium. Did the researchers delve into the diet of the sufferers being researched?

Other authorities suggest that stress or strong emotions can stop the manufacture of hydrochloric acid in the stomach and destroy the Vitamin C reserve in the adrenals within seconds. This in turn means that there are no body acids to dissolve the calcium and thus it piles up; proteins are not digested, toxins accumulate and infection can take hold. Thus illness and ageing are invited.

Now why the accent on the stress factor all of a sudden? It would appear that the healing fraternities are bent on making a solid case for stress in the cause of arthritis. I say they are off beam, but I'm sure that won't stop them. They will bring up more and more reinforcements to prove stress is the guilty culprit . . . and they'll do more and more rigging of statistics. Then soon they will be telling us they have laid arthritis by the heels with their drugs, prosthesis, surgery and manipulation treatment.

Why are the 'healers' doing this? What is the motive behind the facade of stress and emotion? Ah, as Shakespeare might have said, there is the rub!

The medical profession says and has said for centuries that there is no known cause of arthritis and there is no known cure. Righto!

Stress, strain and emotional conditions do not readily respond to treatment but treatments of various sorts must be given. Better still, treatment must be continued 'ad infinitum.' What a beautiful disease from the medical practitioners' standpoint.

The stress, strain and emotions theory will still give them the opportunity to say, "See, we told you all along it has nothing to do with what you eat."

Better still — and here is the trump card — it takes the patient right off the hook and the healer can show great concern and sympathy for the afflicted, saying something like this, "It wasn't your fault. After all, what can you do when you are living in these stressful times? You poor unfortunate person, we will give you one of the newest and best drugs to lighten your load and you'll feel better immediately. Yes, this modern living and the rat race do strange things to human beings."

Contrast this to Tobe's reply to someone complaining about his arthritis problems, which would go something like this, "You like to have your tea and crumpets, coffee, cocktails, cigarettes, bacon and eggs, French fries, and the thousand and one other niceties and pleasantries in the form of processed foods, now don't you? Well, this is the price you pay . . . arthritis or worse! Do you wish to correct your condition? Then start on a diet of raw vegetables, grains, fruits and nuts. Not tomorrow but today!"

In my opinion, arthritis is an earned disease. You do not catch arthritis, you do not have it inflicted upon you, you do not get it by accident and you do not get it through emotional upsets. You get it because over a period of many long years you worked hard at it and earned it by violating nature's laws.

I will grant that stress, strain, tension and emotion can disturb the body's chemistry. Sometimes muscles go into knots, blood circulation is interfered with, blood vessels become constricted, the glandular system malfunctions or the normal hormonal supplies are disturbed. But I contend that a well-nourished, healthy body is in a much better position to withstand the stress and strain . . . in fact, a healthy body can and does stand the strain.

CHAPTER 14

RELIEF OF PAIN

The American Medical Association and the drug corporations, along with the aid of the various research organizations, the Arthritis Foundation and the government, are all out to conquer pain. They have now come up with the belief that pain or suffering is the greatest enemy of mankind and they are going all-out to destroy pain, even if they must kill themselves and everyone else in their campaign to do so.

They have not yet decided how they are going to conquer it but pain is their number one target today. They don't care which drug or how many drugs they use or whether it is done by using surgery, X-rays or radium treatments. Yes, and now they have a new tool — acupuncture, the famed Chinese method of treatment. There are also acupressure, reflexology and zone therapy; all of which are more or less synonymous terms.

Now I want to make it clear that I am all for relieving the pain and suffering of people, no matter what it is that's causing the pain . . . and the most widespread form of pain throughout America today is the pain brought about by arthritis in its many and various forms. However, I have always been a firm believer in cause and effect. Therefore, I maintain that if the cause is removed, the effect or the arthritis pain will slowly but surely disappear — in fact, often quickly.

Even as a boy or a young man, whenever something went wrong with me, I wanted to find out why. When I was told over and over again that my aches were due to growing pains, natural causes or to overtaxed muscles, I had grave doubts as to the veracity of these statements. You see, even early in life I believed in cause and effect.

Now I wonder in my cynicism why the various healing professions are so concerned about relieving pain. Is it because they truly want to ease the suffering of humanity? Or is it because they want to peddle, prescribe or sell a commodity which is both lucrative and continuous?

I suggest their attitude is this. If people have pain and we cannot cure it, we must keep on giving them a pain reliever — be it a drug, placebo, massage, manipulation, therapy or some other form of treatment. Thus, it is easy to understand how a healer with a hundred or so arthritic and other patients coming to see him regularly once a week or once a month could add substantially to his gross dollar intake.

Well, here and now we have hundreds of researchers working on ways and means to relieve pain, with the accent on drugs rather than any other method or means. The use of drugs is by far the easiest and most profitable for the medical profession and the drug manufacturers. Drugs never cure anything but they invariably cause various side-effects which again require medical care and again the use of other drugs. Wow — what a dream of a business or profession! Croesus never had it so good.

People seldom if ever die from the actual pain, especially the pain of arthritis. They suffer, they are uncomfortable and they don't like it, so they keep running back and forth to the doctor. They pay his fee and they take his drugs or medicines. Thus, the doctor is happy, the drug companies are happy and the patient is happy . . . unhappily so.

78

One of the ways that some medical doctors have of relieving pain is to counter the existing pain with pain of another kind. Then in your misery you forget the original pain and concentrate on the secondary pain which was caused for that specific purpose — a counter-irritant, as it is known in the healing circles. Liniments are most frequently used for this purpose.

The healing profession is not overly concerned about the technique or drug used to get rid of the pain as long as the pain subsides and their patient is content. Right now some of the biggest names in the scientific research business are actively working on means and methods of conquering pain.

I just recently read a report entitled, "Pain — The Biggest Problem in U.S. Medicine," and I will quote it in its entirety.

" 'Relief of pain is the greatest unmet need in American medicine today,' says leading pain specialist Dr. Ronald Katz.

" 'Pain is like alcoholism was several years ago — a problem affecting millions but discreetly ignored by society.'

"Dr. Katz ranks pain at the top of the list of problems needing more medical research along with cancer, disease prevention and alcoholism.

" 'The difference is the others are getting lots of publicity and more and more funding. But nobody is doing enough about pain,' he said.

" 'Present research is uncoordinated, fragmented and seriously lacking in funds,' lamented Dr. Katz, who heads a pain treatment clinic at Los Angeles' University of California, where a variety of methods are used, including acupuncture.

" 'There is no one answer to pain . . . no magic pill to solve pain problems.

" 'And I don't see any cure-all for pain in the future — that goes for acupuncture, hypnosis, so-called miracle medications or anything else,' emphasized Dr. Katz, who is also chairman of the department of anesthesiology at the

UCLA School of Medicine.

"He said his pain clinic combines the talents of a number of specialists.

" 'It's a smorgasbord treatment involving such experts as psychiatrists, neurosurgeons, orthopedic surgeons, psychologists, anesthesiologists, anatomists, physiologists and pharmacologists.

" 'We may do a nerve block to remove pain, prescribe medicine, perform acupuncture, hypnotize the patient or teach him to hypnotize himself.

" 'We may refer him to a neurosurgeon or psychiatrist, or do all or just some of these things,' explained Dr. Katz, who said the clinic has 'significantly helped' about half of its patients.

" 'One reason for the percentage not being higher is that many of the patients come to UCLA as a last resort when everything else has failed,' he said.

" 'What is needed is an umbrella agency that will pool all the knowledge being gained from pain research being carried on in various parts of the country.

" 'And more funds are needed for basic research,' insisted Dr. Katz, who also advocates establishing a new field of medical specialization that will focus all its efforts entirely on pain research and the treatment and prevention of it.

" 'Pain is a human misery, a pressing problem for society — and one that deserves far more medical attention.' "

Here is what one great authority on anesthesia and pain, Dr. John J. Bonica, said when he was asked to define pain:

"In my view, pain can be simply defined as an emotional experience either provoked by tissue injury or described by the patient in terms of tissue damage, or both."

Here is how Dr. Bonica describes the origin of pain:

"It works something like this: Information is sent from the body to the brain by sensory nerves which supply every part of the body with nerve endings called 'receptors,' each of

80

which responds specifically to certain stimuli. Some receptors are stimulated by light, others by other special senses, and some by mechanical, temperature or chemical stimulation.

"Each sensory nerve contains thousands of fibers of different size. The large and some small fibers convey such sensations as touch, position sense, and temperature. But some small fibers are used to carry electrical impulses or messages initiated by tissue injury, such as a burn or severe blow. The tissue damage constitutes noxious stimulation which produces impulses that are transmitted to the spinal cord.

"These peripheral fibers are linked to an intricate network of nerve cells in the spinal cord. The point of contact is called a 'synapse' — a very small gap which can be thought of as a gate. Messages jump from one nerve to another through a complex electrochemical process."

It is not my intent to go any further into the mechanics of pain here because this does not come under my competence. I have gone over it with various experts but I am only concerned with getting rid of pain without the use of drugs or palliatives of any kind. I seek total good health for those who read my books and take my advice.

In my lifetime I have suffered the pains of headache, toothache, backache, sciatica, prostate and bladder trouble, cuts, bruises, fractures, neuralgia, tic deloureaux, sprained ankles, chipped bones, etc. so no one need tell me or remind me of how dreadful, how agonizing pain can be. I maintain that no man can think logically or clearly while enduring pain, no man can behave normally, function normally, maneuver normally, act properly, give proper counsel or take matters under consideration or conduct business or attend to his affairs properly while enduring pain.

I can well understand the sufferers, under the duress of pain, seeking anywhere and everywhere for relief. Therefore, I must admit that perhaps pain-relieving drugs do have their

81

place in our way of life ... and perhaps are actually necessary. Please understand that I do not intend to mock either the arthritic sufferer nor the healer who gives him relief. I only bemoan the fact that the indvidual must suffer and the fact that the physician does not give him advice and guidance that will prevent the pain from occurring again and again.

Let me emphasize clearly that I do not believe that drugs, shots, tranquilizers, narcotics and surgery are the real answer to pain. One may get temporary relief this way but he may also end up in worse trouble than the original problem.

What makes matters worse is the fact that when you are in pain and suffering, you want instant relief ... you don't want to wait for an hour or two hours or until tomorrow or next week. You want relief now and you are ready and willing to accept whatever or whoever promises immediate results.

Granted, the medical profession does know how to relieve pain. If you are suffering pain, a shot or one of many drugs will make you totally insensible to your pain. Of course, it will have done nothing to correct the condition causing the pain but when you are suffering, you are not concerned about that. You just want to get some relief and a medical man can do that better than any other person on earth.

So I do not blame the average individual who is suffering from pain for accepting whatever is offered by the practitioner. Pain and suffering drive a man to unbelievable decisions and therefore a man or a person who is suffering is concerned only with the immediate relief from his suffering. However, I contend that the accent should be on finding the causative factors and eliminating them. Thus, no cause, no pain.

CHAPTER 15

THE MEDICAL PROFESSION'S ANSWER

I suggest that it is scandalous for the American Medical Association, the Arthritis Foundation and other money-collecting foundations interested in arthritis, as well as the aspirin companies and the drug corporations, to keep more than 25,000,000 suffering souls in bondage. Yes, they keep their victims shackled to a devious drug cycle and in a state of semi-consciousness or tranquilization. I say that the truth is not told just so they can continue to extract billions of dollars annually from these sufferers.

Now it is bad enough that they extract this money from these people but, even worse, they often inflict more horrible suffering upon them with cortisone and other treatments. With the tacit admission that they do not know the cause nor the cure of arthritis, the medical profession logically rules itself out as a means of cure or positive corrective help to arthritic sufferers. Giving various drugs and treatment for palliation of their suffering only causes or contributes to other diseases and conditions, most of which are more serious and more deadly. These are known as iatrogenic diseases.

In Taber's Cyclopedic Medical Dictionary, under "Iatrogenic disorder" we read: "An abnormal mental or physical condition induced in a patient by effects of treatment by a physician or surgeon. Term implies that such effects could have been avoided by proper and judicious care on the part of the physician."

Then under "Iatrogeny," it says, "Abnormal state or condition induced by a physician."

It is generally accepted that an iatrogenic disease is caused by the use of drugs as prescribed by a physician. There are virtually tens of thousands of drugs that no one knows much about, especially the side-effects. Well, it is these side-effects that I specifically label as iatrogenic diseases.

I note that physicians frequently suggest plenty of bed rest for arthritic patients. Of course, here the medical profession is reverting to one of their old, time-worn practices. Perhaps it is true that in many cases bed rest will lessen pain, but to suggest that bed rest is a cure for arthritis is nothing short of ridiculous.

It was about 40 years ago that it first dawned upon medical practitioners that perhaps rest was not the great benefactor that they had formerly believed it to be. A few experiments crept in which indicated this to be true and now more experiments have been done and it has been positively proven that bed rest, even for broken limbs, is not in the patient's best interest. Most medical men have realigned themselves but many of them are still practising this antiquated bed rest means of treatment for practically every condition.

The best medical and surgical treatment in the world for hernia is practised right in the City of Toronto at the Shouldice Clinic and they do not keep you in bed even after surgery.

Of course, bed rest has been the stand-by of the medical profession since time immemorial . . . and perhaps with good reason. Statistics prove clearly that approximately 85% of all illnesses will clear up or disappear on their own, without any form of treatment. Therefore, if the doctor puts you to bed and does not even give you any medicine at all, the chances are greatly in your favor that you will soon recover. Then the doctor can take credit for the cure.

Maybe there is also some good sound logic in this bed rest practice because when you are resting in bed, you cannot be out carousing, boozing and in other ways forcing insults upon your troubled body. In this light perhaps bed rest is an advantage, but in my humble opinion, bed rest is the last thing in the world that might benefit an arthritic sufferer.

Exercise is also used in the treatment of arthritis and many other conditions. In fact, there are few conditions where exercise will not benefit the individual, especially one whose occupation is sedentary and does not allow much physical labor. Of course, exercise is an alternate for physical work and some of the violent exercises that I have seen done are much more strenuous than actual physical work.

Every morning I do about 15 minutes of exercises, but I assure you that I would much rather chop wood for one hour and I am sure it would do me more good. Occasionally I do chop wood and I prefer it by far but I always have a heavy load of desk work to do. I just don't have time to change my clothes and go down to the wood shed and chop wood for an hour or so every morning. However, I assure you that the 15 minutes of strenuous exercises that I do are much harder on me and more distasteful than one hour of wood chopping which I would enjoy.

The benefits of exercise can never be exaggerated and there is no doubt about it that exercise for arthritis victims can be a tremendous boon, but while I am totally in favor of exercise, I maintain that exercise in itself is not as effectual as exercise in combination with a change of diet and mode of living. Combine good eating habits, good living habits and sound health principles with physical work or exercise and there you have the most powerful weapon in dealing with arthritis or any other disease.

I presume that you have heard the old adage, "A man

who is his own doctor has a fool for a physician."

Well, I disagree with that statement and recommend that each man be his own doctor — assuming that he has normal intelligence and is willing to ask questions, read and investigate. Judging from the arthritics that I have seen — and I have seen virtually thousands of people suffering from various forms of arthritis — those enjoying or undergoing medical attention were almost invariably worse off than those who were treating themselves.

Please understand that the medical men go on their merry way treating arthritics with thousands of different drugs and by various other means, including surgery . . . at the same time singing the refrain that they do not know the cause and they do not know the cure. Does this make any sense to you?

My advice, strict and to the point, is to learn to live and depend upon your own intelligence, your willingness to learn and your will power. Will power is vitally important, so you will not indulge in foods and a way of life that can and do contribute to the cause of arthritis. The only things the doctor has to offer you are aspirin, the gold treatment, surgery, cortisone and other drugs — all of which do more harm than good. So I say with all my heart, "You are better off to treat yourself!"

Let it be understood very clearly that while arthritis cannot be cured or even stopped by medical means, it can be cured and stopped by other means. Actually what the medical profession means but does not spell out clearly is that arthritis cannot be cured by drugs, surgery, X-ray and radium. However, in America today there are thousands of people who have suffered from arthritis but who do not suffer today. Their condition is clearly under control or has completely disappeared due to other than medical means.

Here and now it might be interesting to ask the question, "What happens when the doctor gets arthritis?"

Well, it so happens that there is a case on record, of a doctor who had arthritis. This medical doctor, of course, followed his colleagues' advice and from his story we read:

"Weeks and months passed, and with them, therapeutic efforts which were as ingenious as they were futile. One which still stands out in my memory with clarity and horror was the intravenous administration of typhoid vaccine. The first dose gave a most gratifying reaction, a rapid febrile response to 106 degrees and a chill which literally snapped one of the side rails of my bed. Unfortunately, I had failed to place any shock-absorbing substance between my teeth, and later inspection revealed the enamel chipped from two incisors. The result of this drastic procedure was nothing short of astounding; during the following forty-eight hours I was completely free of joint pain and had normal mobility for the first time since the onset of my illness. However, a prompt return to the preshock status constituted the bitterest disappointment of my life, and subsequent injections with larger dosage failed to evoke a similar reaction or improvement. In this day of enthusiastic and sometimes ill-advised treatment with cortisone, I can very easily identify myself with those previously hopeless patients who have a good initial response and a subsequent exacerbation. . . .

"My regimen in the sanatorium was one which treated not only the arthritis, but the man. A carefully planned diet, high in protein, minerals and vitamins, began to replace the forty pounds which I had lost during the initial phase of my illness. Graduated plaster splints coaxed my wrists and ankles into reasonably good alignment. The application of a bewildering variety of physiotherapeutic measures, ranging from paraffin packs to warm pool exercises, began to stretch the adhesions in many of my immobile joints. General and localized heliotherapy, rigidly controlled by a stop watch, stimulated my peripheral circulation and atrophied skin. One of the many ingenious and pain-saving devices, the importance of which every arthritic will acclaim, was the provision of a built-up lavatory seat which eliminated the necessity of flexing inflamed knee joints. Often did I bless the unknown inventor of this gadget, which spared me the final indignity of having to be assisted on and off the throne! . . .

"I do remember, however, that the hot, swollen, and tender joints in the early weeks of the disease were not materially eased by the administration of large doses of aspirin and sodium salicylate. The net result of this type of medication was so much gastric distress that I discontinued it of my own volition, preferring the pain to this alternative. Possibly the buffered preparations now in use may be more tolerable in this respect. Codeine, sparingly used at the peak of the inflammatory process, was much more helpful, and the side effects were negligible in the small doses employed. However, in my experience, analgesic drug therapy was of relatively little help for long-term relief. Major amelioration was obtained from the judicious use of proper immobilization and from certain forms of the application of heat. The wearing of properly angulated, light plaster splints rather promptly afforded relief from both the dull, nagging pain associated with the weight of an extremity and the lightning-sharp twinges caused by muscle spasm. Comforting heat, one of nature's oldest remedies, did not require such complicated gadgets as diathermy and short-wave machines; although these were tried and soon discarded. The application of large, warm, moist packs was very soothing to large joints, while paraffin packs, as hot as could be tolerated, were most practical for small joints of the hands and feet. . . .

"Further medical care, restricted practice and frequent vacations resulted in continued improvement and increasing strength, but it eventually became obvious that I probably would never have total restoration of joint and muscle function. It was at this point that, aided by the wisdom of one of the great men of internal medicine, I made a decision which I have never regretted. 'Doctor,' he said, 'you are a very fortunate man. Your fate might have been different. You can still practice your profession, but it must be under conditions which will give the greatest possible assurance against another relapse. You know what those conditions are. Good luck.'

"During my long illness I had been told that, contrary to tradition, I was considered a good patient who swallowed his prescriptions faithfully. It was therefore consistent that I accepted this latest advice and again turned to the West. This time it was a happier expedition; I was able to drive my car and to take my family with me. While I was casting about for the type of medical work which would be compatible with my residual disability, a position on the staff of a tuberculosis sanatorium was offered. It immediately became obvious that this presented the ideal solution to my problem. The relatively sheltered life in an institutional environment made it possible for me to follow, at least in principle, the controlled regimen of the ex-tuberculosis physicians who were my colleagues. Undisturbed nights of sleep, regularity of working hours and meals, a midday rest period and relative freedom from undue physical exertion were major factors in helping to husband my meager physical resources and to avoid the causes of reactivation.

"For thirteen years I have been able to continue, in various capacities, this quiet but satisfying existence. My labors have been unspectacular but rewarding. Such pleasures as music, reading, bridge, swimming and motor trips are adequate substitutes for more strenuous amusements. When my joints are particularly comfortable, I may even feel devilish enough to indulge in a restrained game of ping-pong or a round of miniature golf. But by the same token I have a very legitimate excuse to avoid carrying wood for the fireplace or mowing the lawn.

"If, as an eminent expert has stated, rheumatoid arthritis

89

usually burns itself out in fifteen years, the remainder of my life will be pure profit."

Now that you have the story of the best that the great, all powerful and noble medical profession can offer for arthritis, are you ready to try nature's way? Are you ready to try a raw food diet and a proper natural way of life? By this means not only will you control the disease but you will regain your health and mobility, too, provided you have not waited too long. However, at any stage it is worth a try, because you have everything to gain and absolutely nothing to lose . . . except your pain and crippling!

CHAPTER 16

ARTIFICIAL JOINTS

From what I have learned, it appears that the first surgery on arthritic joints was performed at the beginning of this century and in those days the operations most certainly were not accepted or considered safe and legitimate as a means of treating people with arthritic problems. It has only been in the last 20 or 25 years that surgery for arthritis has been looked upon with anything like favor.

Furthermore, in the early days of surgery for arthritis they felt that the arthritis had to subside before surgery could be attempted. Today, they consider it safe to operate when the arthritic condition is virulent and active. Not only do they replace various pieces of bone structure and joints, but they go much further than that and remove painful and inflamed tissue, too.

If you will check the records you will find that surgery for arthritis is becoming more and more common and I predict that some day it will become the most common form of surgery practised in America. Of course the reason for my prediction is that there are more people in America suffering from arthritis than from any other disease.

From what I have read and judging from medical-surgical

opinion, it appears to be fairly easy to replace a joint in the human body. However, I do not consider it so easy to make that synthetic joint function properly in relation to other normal joints. But at the present time it appears that physicians, surgeons, physiotherapists and patients are all combining efforts to make arthritic surgery a practical, functional operation.

Now I would like to outline the various kinds of present day arthritic surgery. There may be many more but these are the ones that I have become acquainted with so far:

Arthroplasty is the kind of surgery that molds a new joint to replace the diseased one and this is attached to the ends of the bone that forms the old joint. Various metals are used to replace bony parts of the joint.

Then there is arthroclasia which is artificial breaking of an ankylosed joint usually performed on the knee or the hip and sometimes on the wrist because the hand is no longer functional.

Arthrodesis is the surgical fixation of a joint.

Next is synovectomy which is the removal of swollen, enlarged or diseased synovial membrane. They also remove any loose pieces of tissue that may be hampering or locking the joint. While synovectomy is most frequently performed at the knee, it is also done at many other joints. This type of surgery is also performed where the tendon sheaths are inflamed.

Then there is the surgery known as contraction release or freeing the contraction. The contracting tissue that surrounds the deformity is freed by the surgeon, thus enabling the joint to function again.

Then there is osteotomy, which is surgery performed on the bones around the joint where the joints' surfaces have been injured or destroyed by the disease in active form. This condition is found specifically in osteoarthritis of the hip and the hip needs to be realigned.

They now perform biopsies in arthritis, too. The surgeon considers this to be a most simple operation, wherein he removes a piece of the tissue for diagnosis.

Articles glorifying surgery for arthritis continue to crop up in the medical magazines and medically-sponsored magazines, as well as other magazines. For example, here is the introductory paragraph from an article in the Family Health magazine, entitled "New Victories in the Fight Against Arthritis":

"Now, thousands of arthritis sufferers can get a new lease on life as pioneering surgeons perfect artificial joints and reasearchers develop drugs to fight the nation's No. 1 crippler. Even the ultimate goal — prevention — is in sight."

Then they usually tell about some famous men who have had artificial joints put into their bodies. Is is said they suffer no more, can do their work and perform their normal duties . . . everything is great and wonderful.

This one particular article quotes Eugene Ormandy, the 73-year-old Director of the Philadelphia Orchestra, as saying, "It is such a wonderful feeling to walk once again to the podium without pain or embarrassment."

Frankly, being the most doubting of doubting Thomases, I would like to hear these words today from Mr. Ormandy's own lips, man to man.

This reminds me of the great to-do and publicity given that man in South Africa — Blaiberg, I believe it was — who had a heart-transplant and later was doing so wonderfully well that he was attending parties, having a good time and doing splendidly. Then eventually he died and he left a note telling how he had suffered every second of his life after the surgery. He said it was agony for him and he had wished he were dead many times. This story was corroborated by his family.

Now I suspect — in fact, I am reasonably sure — that this is the case with many people who have these artificial joints. I assume that they suffer, too, and have to take drugs every day of their lives to relieve pain and prevent infection. The body's immunological system will be fighting the invader with every breath and every beat of the heart and they will have to take drugs to offset this rejection also.

I do not suggest that all arthritis surgery is a failure or that all patients suffer the agonies of the damned for the rest of their lives. However, I do suggest that you don't count on surgery to be the answer to all your prayers . . . for surgery is not as yet an exact, predictable science.

I say to eat right and live right. Then, even with advanced arthritis you can avoid or lessen your aches, pains and crippling. So instead of taking the grave risk of surgery, start protecting yourself today.

I would like to quote here a few more paragraphs from this same article, "New Victories in the Fight Against Arthritis":

"To the recipients, these artificial joints are indeed a 'new lease on life.' Take, for example, Mrs. Sally Smith, a 39-year-old Cleveland housewife who has become increasingly crippled from rheumatoid arthritis over the last 15 years. The onset of her disease, when she was 24, could be described as classical, according to Dr. Alan H. Wilde, a specialist in arthritis surgery at Cleveland Clinic. She suffered a loss of weight, fatigue, frequent high temperatures, and, as she remembers, 'My joints were so stiff and sore, I could hardly get out of bed in the morning.'

"As the joints in her wrists and fingers became more swollen and painful, she sought medical help, and rheumatoid arthritis was diagnosed. In this stage of the disease, the synovial membrane — the lining of the fibrous tissues around the joint — becomes inflamed and thickened and begins to grow. At the same time, more synovial fluid, the substance that lubricates the joint, accumulates, leading to painful swelling. As the disease advances, the cartilage and bone become eroded, and the fibrous tissues may be replaced by bone. This results in possible dislocation or in a solid, fused joint, incapable of normal movement.

"In Mrs. Smith's case, the disease quickly spread to her knees, feet, shoulders and right hip. 'It seemed to let up when I was pregnant,' she said, 'but it always came back, worse than before, after each baby was born.' Many women report these periods of remission during pregnancy, but they seldom last. Since arthritis is a disease of ups and downs, there are mysterious calm periods when it seems to fade away, only to return with a severe attack that leaves the sufferer more crippled than ever. Over the years, Mrs. Smith became increasingly disabled, depressed and ineffective as a wife and mother to her three children, now aged 12, eight and six.

" 'I had to use a walker or a wheel-chair,' she recalls. 'The pain in my hip never went away, and I seldom had more than an hour or two of uninterrupted sleep. I was allergic to the gold treatments, and I couldn't take cortisone either. I seemed to live on aspirin. Life was pretty grim for all of us, especially my children.'

"Early this year, Mrs. Smith entered Cleveland Clinic for a total hip replacement — the same operation Mr. Ormandy had. Up until 18 months ago, only about 5,000 such operations had been performed in this country. But the hip replacement has become today's fastest growing field of orthopedic surgery, with up to two million potential candidates. Experts estimate that 20,000 - 25,000 will be performed this year alone.

95

"The simple ball-and-socket construction of the hip, its size (the largest joint in the body), and the surrounding mass of muscle tissue make it a prime candidate for replacement with a prosthesis. Hip operations, using a variety of mechanical joint substitutes, have been done for 40 years, but with a high number of failures. Today's growing number of successes are attributed to engineering advances — a new metal-and-plastic prosthesis developed by England's Dr. John Charnley and his discovery that it can be cemented into place with methyl methacrylate, an acrylic glue used by dentists. Before, the artificial joints were held in place by screws, which often worked loose after a year or two.

"In the 90-minute 'total hip' operation, the head of the femur (the thigh bone) is removed and replaced with a metal ball attached to a shaft that is cemented into the bone. The socket is then hollowed out to make room for a plastic socket, made of a high-density polyethylene, which is cemented into place. So far, this plastic socket seems to wear well, and does not present the lubrication problems encountered with the earlier metal sockets. However, Dr. Charnley cautions that it might eventually wear thin, especially in the younger, more active patients, and have to be replaced. There are other complications — infection is a prime danger, and extra precautions must be taken, both with antibiotic therapy and in operating-room procedures."

If they tell you they are winning the war against arthritis and they are conquering it, as the heading of the article indicates, why did this woman have to go through all those years of agony?

Also, please note that, by their own admission, "Hip operations, using a variety of mechanical joint substitutes, have been done for 40 years, but with a high number of failures." Well, I must say that I have been around for almost

70 years and I have never known of one 'mechanical joint' that worked properly or without pain and suffering.

The Arthritis Foundation is the fountainhead which sponsored a fairly recent meeting in Dallas where more than 1200 scientists, doctors and press members gathered to hear 154 papers describing scientific advances on various forms of arthritis. It was the largest meeting of arthritis specialists that has ever been held in the United States . . . and, no doubt, one could say in the world as well.

Those 1,200 doctors, scientists and newsmen in Dallas were there for one purpose and one purpose only and that was to make arthritis pay more money. They weren't concerned about the suffering people. If they were, they would tell them the truth, "Give up all the junk food you are enjoying, go on a raw food diet and you won't need drugs, surgery or replacement parts . . . and your suffering will end."

I contend that the medical profession brought surgery and replacement parts into the act when they realized the dismal failure they were experiencing in the treatment of arthritis with drugs. They tell us today that if drugs fail, surgery often helps by providing artificial joints. They say this when almost everyone knows, and they admit, that drugs have been a total failure.

When a limb has been damaged beyond repair and there is suffering and agony, surgery would appear to be the only way out. However, many people accept surgery or are talked into surgery when it is not really necessary. It is this type of situation that I am referring to at this time. I just want to point out to you that all is not rosy and bright for those who have this type of surgery performed.

I want to bring to your attention this reference that was made in the Medical Post of April 29, 1975, to 'geometric' total knee surgery and I quote:

"The first 100 'geometric' total knees done at the Cleveland Clinic have now been followed up for two years.

"A report to the American Academy of Orthopedic Surgeons here indicates this new prosthesis generally gives 90 per cent good results — at least in the short term.

"But there are still concerns.

"One involves the question of wear. Cement debris drops into or onto the weight-bearing plastic lower component and this can cause havoc.

"And the loosening at the bone/cement interface is 'disquieting.'

"The total knee is not as spectacular from another point of view as its senior cousin, the total hip.

" 'You never quite see the elation from patients with a total knee that you do in patients with a total hip,' says Dr. Alan H. Wilde, head of the section of rheumatoid surgery at the clinic. 'I'm not quite sure why this should be so . . . whether in hip disease the patient is relieved of more pain or what. You never seem to get the patients coming back jumping with joy as you do in the hip. But it is a good operation . . . much better than anything else we had to offer before.' "

Now you will note that they are elated over the success they have achieved with hip surgery and consider it a masterpiece.

I would like to refer to another article referring to prosthetic surgery which appeared in the Medical Post of May 27, 1975 and the headline reads: "Two Main Reasons for Prosthetic Hip Failures."

"Mechanical failures of total hip prostheses are showing up more frequently — particularly fractures of the stem of the femoral component.

"According to Dr. Scales one clinic in Munich amassed

50 cases of broken femoral stem. Another in Milan had 30 cases. All fractures were in the stem. None seem to break through the neck.

" 'We have taken 17 of these broken prostheses and tried to reconstruct what happened. The story embraces a whole spectrum of problems. Some of the stems failed in a few months while others took years. It appears the heavier the patient the worse the risk.' . . .

"Dr. Keith Markolf (PhD) an assistant professor of biomechanics, bioengineering and orthopedics at the University of California at Los Angeles said most of the failures he had investigated were caused by metal fatigue.

" 'They begin when the stem bends. The stem is supported and typically a small crack will appear on the lateral surface and grow through a cross section until the remaining metal is no longer strong enough to hold up.' "

I would like to bring to your attention part of an article on arthritis that appeared in Northern Neighbors giving some information received from Dr. S. I. Surgeyev of the U.S.S.R.:

"In recent years, doctors have paid much attention to transplants of organs (heart, kidney, bone, skin, etc.). Sad to say, our bodies reject transplants from other bodies; to make transplants 'take', chemicals were developed which stop the body from rejecting the 'invader'.

"But even sadder: sometimes the chemicals help the body to accept a transplant, but at the same time they may lead to development of cancer."

So I am asking the question, "Can these hip, knee and other prosthetic replacement parts result in cancer? Would it be a matter of exchanging arthritis for cancer?" If it is, it wouldn't be a very profitable exchange, would it?

I would like to quote now from the Medical Post of April 1, 1975, from an article concerning infection after joint replacement:

"Both patients and doctors should note that after total joint surgery any infection of other systems should not be taken lightly.

" 'If a patient with a total hip develops an infection it should be stamped on quickly,' says Dr. Philip Wilson.

"In an interview Dr. Wilson, surgeon in chief and professor of orthopedic surgery at the Hospital for Special Surgery in New York City, said this lesson had been learned years ago by heart surgeons who were implanting heart valves.

"Now it is time to get the same message across to orthopedists.

" 'And any surgeon doing implant work should make sure his patient knows of the dangers.'

"Dr. Wilson was senior author in a paper presented to this year's annual meeting of the American Academy of Orthopedic Surgeons. His co-authors were Drs. Tyrone D. Artz, now of Wichita Clinic, Wichita, Joseph Macys, Eduardo A. Salvati, and Bernard Jacobs all from Dr. Wilson's department in New York.

"The team reported four cases in which a total hip suffered an hematogenous metastatic infection.

"They add that there are only scattered reports in the orthopedic literature which mention this hazard. For example, Charnley — the father of the total hip — has only published one case in which infection in a hip was seen after his patient developed septic pharyngitis.

"The four cases the NYC surgeons have encountered each occurred from three to 39 months after hip surgery which had no immediate infectious complications."

They tell us further that surgical replacement of various joints has increased tenfold in the last ten years. They claim that almost 40,000 Americans each year are enabled to walk again with artificial hip joints.

From an article in Time Magazine of March 18, 1974, we read:

"A man of many artificial parts was lawyer Frank Tull. His teeth had been fashioned for him and fitted to his jaws by a doctor of dental surgery . . . He had a silver plate in his skull to guard a hole from which a brain tumor had been removed. One of his legs was made of metal and fibre; it took the place of the flesh-and-blood leg his mother had given him in her womb . . . In his left arm, a platinum wire took the place of the humerus . . . One hundred years after he died they opened up his coffin. All they found were strings and wires.

"In 1935, when author Charles Finney created him as a character in the novel *The Circus of Dr. Lao*, Frank Tull was considered to be, at most, the product of a fertile imagination. Yet, less than 40 years later, the concept of semi-artificial man no longer seems as far-fetched. Though modern medicine has yet to produce a real-life counterpart of television's *Six Million Dollar Man* it has developed workable replacements for many important body parts, and is steadily moving toward the day when hospitals may well have to follow the lead of auto-repair shops and add spare-parts departments to their facilities.

"Man has been replacing damaged portions of his body with artificial parts for centuries. Peg legs have been used since 600 B.C., and metal hands since the 16th century. Boston Silversmith Paul Revere was well known for the quality of false teeth he fashioned long before his midnight message to Massachusetts' minutemen. But today's many and various replacements made of such space-age materials as Teflon, the non-stick plastic, and pyrolytic carbon, a diamond-hard substance, are far more sophisticated. Unlike

101

earlier devices which were worn outside the body and usually removed at night, they are true replacements, designed to be implanted permanently and to duplicate, if not actually improve upon nature."

Yes, records clearly indicate that arthritic surgery is becoming very popular. Whether this is due to good results achieved or to the great promotional effort that is being put forth by the various organizations, I don't know. But from the bottom of my heart, I hope that the surgeons are achieving great and lasting results.

CHAPTER 17

CHIROPRACTORS AND ARTHRITIS

Dragging the chiropractors into this book on arthritis may seem a bit strange but when I get through with this chapter you will probably understand my reason.

During most of my youth and early adult life I suffered off and on from various aches and pains ... but in spite of those occasional aches and pains, I was considered a very healthy person. I had aches and pains in my shoulders, in my arms and occasionally in my legs but whenever I had the opportunity to talk to a doctor, he assured me that I did not require any medical attention. He would always pass it off by saying, "Ah, those are just growing pains. You are as healthy as a man can be. Everyone gets an ache or a pain now and then!"

Finally, after I had read and studied nutrition thoroughly, I realized that this was pure hyperbole and a healthy person should not have these aches and pains. A completely healthy, well adjusted person with a well nourished body knows no aches or pains of any kind.

When I first had a really bad bout of back pain, which in those days they called lumbago or sciatica, someone suggested that I should go to a chiropractor. Well, one day when I was in real agony, I did visit one of these manipulators and, let's face it, I did get relief. In fact, I walked into the chiropractor's office all bent over and crippled up, so to speak, and I walked out straight.

However, this good thing did not last and in a day or two I was right back where I was before . . . but I must admit that the chiropractor did give me temporary relief. Furthermore, chiropractors gave me relief on many other occasions as well . . . without the use of drugs.

I recall some years ago when I had an exceptionally bad bout of this condition — in no way am I calling it arthritis but I had pains in my back, in my legs and in my arms — I was advised to go to a highly esteemed masseur. I went to him and he gave me a series of treatments. I must admit that the treatments surely made me feel good but it was a long drawn-out affair and the pains did recur. Sometimes they would be less severe and sometimes they would be more severe . . . but, I repeat, the treatments were pleasant and they did relax me and make me feel much better at the time.

Through the years I was led to believe that the medical doctors could not do much for you when it came to back pains, as most of them suffered from such aches and pains themselves. Thus, I had no alternative but to go to the chiropractor or the masseur . . . and this was practically the story of my life.

Then my wife became afflicted. Her condition worsened and worsened until she was hobbling around and she developed curvature of the spine. She tried various chiropractors and masseurs and they did give her some comfort but she was becoming a cripple.

Her father finally decided to take a hand in the affair and he took her to Toronto where she began the round of the medical specialists. They told her the same story — that there was little or nothing they could do — until one day she came across a specialist who said he could fix her up. This seemed like very, very good news to my wife and her father. This doctor said, "Here is what we have to do. You come in and I will break your spine where the curvature is and then I will rebuild it. You will be in a cast for about six months."

Then my wife asked the big question, "Will that straighten out my spine?"

He said, "Yes, I guarantee that this will straighten out your spine. I may have to fuse it but I guarantee it will be straight."

My wife decided she would go in for surgery. I kept my nose clean. I had done all I knew and I did not know anything, but I certainly did not approve of having one's spine broken and then being put in a cast for six months or more. However, my wife and her father had made the decision about this, so what could I say?

In any event, before they went ahead with this surgery, a friend of the family suggested that there was another doctor who was getting fairly good results with a new gimmick. Well, they went to see this man, who was also a medical doctor in Toronto, and he advised them not to go through with the surgery. He said that from his experience surgery did not bring very good results and in many cases the pain was still there when they were finished . . . with a fused spine, to boot.

My father-in-law asked, "What do you offer?"

He said, "I offer a very simple treatment. Take your daughter home and put her to bed, but put a sheet of 3/4 inch or 1 inch plywood under the mattress. She must sleep on a firm bed."

Remember, this was a medical doctor in good standing, yet that was his total therapy. She did as he suggested and every day I would check her spine with a yardstick to see if it was straightening out. Lo and behold, in a matter of three weeks her spine was straight.

Now I strongly urge you to believe what I am telling you because, I swear, it is absolutely true. I used to check her spine with that yardstick every morning and then report to her. After about the second week it showed great improvement and, as I stated previously, at the end of the third week it had straightened right out.

I have known many people who were advised to go in for surgery and have their spines fused. If I knew in advance what they intended to have done, I would warn them and tell them this story — but very few ever believed me. The surgeon and the doctor suggested they have the operation and they did. Afterwards, they had fused spines and couldn't bend properly — and most of them still had just as much pain as before.

I must say that when my wife consulted the chiropractor in our town, who came to our home to give her treatments, he did help her to feel much better. There are no if's, and's or but's about it . . . he gave her relief and he did help her to recover.

Now I want to make it clear that I have no specific love for any one healer over another. To be frank, I have friends and I mean good, dear friends who are medical doctors, I have dear, close friends who are chiropractors and I have some good friends who are naturopathic physicians. I also have very good friends who practice some of the other healing arts.

When it comes to healers, I show no preference except that I think a naturopathic physician is less apt to do you harm than any of the other healers and a chiropractor is less apt to do you harm than a knife-wielding, drug-dispensing, X-ray-taking, radium-shooting medical doctor. I do not consider healers to be benefactors of mankind. In fact, to the contrary, in general I think they do mankind more harm than good . . . and I say that seriously and with the full realization of what I am saying.

When I was suffering quite badly one time, I went to a chiropractic doctor — an old timer in Niagara Falls, Ontario — and after a couple of treatments that didn't do me any good he decided that he had best put me in traction, which he did. Of course, traction means that they lay you on a board or an operating table and tie weights to your legs or to your feet and they actually stretch your legs and spine. I understand medical doctors also practise this "bed of Procrustes"* stunt.

Well, I thought I had had pain with my backache, lumbago, sciatica or whatever but, man, that traction really gave me pain! It was sheer agony but I must admit that after a couple of treatments the backache did seem to be lessening. The traction was absolute agony so my original back pains seemed small in comparison.

Well, after three or four of these treatments, the chiropractor discovered that my left leg was shorter than my right. He checked it again and again and he said, "Yes, your left leg is about a quarter of an inch shorter than the right one, so you will have to wear a lift in your left shoe for the remainder of your life."

Then I went on my merry way and as I was driving home from Niagara Falls I thought to myself, "Tobe, as a young boy you ran like the wind and were a champion runner — you could outrun any kid in the area. You played baseball — and you were a darn good ball player. You could run the bases like crazy and as an outfielder or a shortstop, you could move around as well as anyone who ever walked. Besides this, you played basketball for years and you skated and played

*Procrustes was a Greek bandit.

hockey, too. Why should someone who went through all those years with a pair of agile, normal legs and body suddenly turn up with one leg shorter than the other?"

I chided myself, "Come off it, Tobe. This is insanity!"

I took the lift out of my shoe and threw it away. I don't know where it went as I threw it far . . . and I never went back to that chiropractor again!

One thing I have against chiropractors is this traction treatment that they use on many of their patients or should I say, victims. Well, I think those chiropractors should be hung by their heels in their "traction" for this type of practice, if they are still doing it. This is only my personal opinion.

I would like to quote from an article in The Medical Letter of February 14, 1975, under heading, "Low-Back Pain":

"It is generally agreed that in acute low-back pain, with severe muscle spasm and tilting of the trunk, the patient is best treated with complete bed rest, heat and analgesics. There is only one controlled clinical trial of traction in chronic low-back pain — a report by H. Weber (J. Oslo City Hospital., 23:167, 1973) on 72 patients with radiating pains and neurological signs. The patients were separated into two groups: those to whom traction was applied, and those given simulated traction. The physicians who evaluated the effects did not know which a given patient had received. Traction had no beneficial effect compared to simulated traction. Many orthopedists, physiotherapists and neurosurgeons believe that recumbency reduces the forces acting on the lumbar disk more than any form of traction."

Another thing I have against chiropractors is that if you go to a chiropractor for treatment, you will almost invariably be X-rayed. I think every chiropractor in America who can beg, borrow or steal the money has an X-ray machine . . . and, boy, that X-ray machine is better than having a permit to print money. Chiropractors even go a few steps further than the medical men, who only X-ray certain limited areas of the body, because chiropractors take X-rays of your whole body . . . and they take them as if they were going out of style.

When I confronted two or three chiropractors about this outrage, as I call it, they told me it was necessary in order to protect themselves against malpractice suits. Just how or why whole body X-rays would help the doctor in the event of a malpractice suit is never explained, but that's the answer they give. I feel that they say this as a 'cover-up.'

Now I do not know whether the chiropractor was taught this gimmick at college or not but, anyway, I got a variety of answers from different chiropractors when I posed this question with a twinkle in my eye, "It isn't to make money, is it? You don't make money on these X-rays, do you?"

In any event, I consider taking X-rays of the human body to be a harmful, body-destroying practice. I believe that even the smallest or shortest X-ray is harmful and the large X-rays that the chiropractor takes can be downright deadly. Yes, I feel sure chiropractors are doing irreparable harm to their patients by the indiscriminate use of X-rays.

If I were a chiropractic patient and I developed cancer a few years after treatment, I would say to the chiropractor, "I am going to sue you because I think this practice of shooting X-rays of the whole body is criminal and I think you caused or contributed to my present condition."

This chapter will not make me very popular with the chiropractic profession, I'm sure. No doubt, I will be as popular with the "chiros" as I am with the "medics." However, it is not that I love chiropractors less but that I love the truth more.

CHAPTER 18

SEX AND ARTHRITIS

Just recently I read where a medical doctor advised against sex for anyone with arthritis. He believes sex to be a factor in the cause of arthritis. However, another famous doctor advises the opposite and I will quote from Dr. Reuben's book, "Everything You Always Wanted to Know About Sex, But Were Afraid to Ask":

"What about people with arthritis?"

"As time passes almost everyone develops occasional aches and pains in their bones and joints. Sometimes the discomfort gets to the point where intercourse and the associated movement can cause pain. This is the worst possible reason to cut back on sexual activity. For most forms of arthritis, frequent mild exercise is beneficial. What better way is there to exercise mildly than in the comfort and privacy of one's bed with an attractive sexual partner?

"But there is even a better reason than that. All the glands in the body are interconnected and ruled by the master gland, the pituitary. Since the testicles in the male and the ovaries in the female are affected by sexual activity, the message is sent back to the pituitary at the base of the brain. This stimulates, in turn, the thyroid and the adrenal glands to

111

increase their production of cortisone and tends to alleviate the symptoms of arthritis."

"You mean sex is good for arthritis?"

"In a sense, yes. For a long time doctors have known that there is much less arthritis among those who remain sexually active. They used to think that only those who somehow were spared the crippling effects of this disease were able to keep having intercourse. Now, hormone studies have proved that it is sexual activity itself which helps protect those beyond middle age from the degenerative changes of this condition."

So there you have it. We have one physician who claims that sex on the part of the male is the cause of arthritis and he says, "I advise complete sexual abstinence until a cure is completed and moderation for the future," and another who says just the opposite.

My personal experience has been that even when one is suffering excruciating pain, one can still perform the sex act. I can recall many occasions in my lifetime when I was suffering pain — specifically back pain or pain that used to be called 'sciatica.' Although I could hardly endure the pain all through the day or get a decent night's sleep, when the body felt the need of sexual intercourse, the pain seemed to subside or totally disappear. Now, I am talking about something that I actually experienced so in this regard I can speak with actual authority.

When the desire for sexual relations came on, the pain totally disappeared. Whereas 5 or 10 minutes earlier I would not have dared to stoop or bend, suddenly I could do all of the maneuvers and functions necessary to perform the sex act in what I believe to be an absolutely normal manner. However, after the completion of the performance, say a few minutes later, the pain slowly but definitely returned with its

112

full vigor. I had quite a time trying to explain this rather embarrassing or paradoxical situation to my sexual partner.

The conclusion that I reached at that time, after thinking things over, was that the sex urge was so powerful that it shut off the pain-causing mechanism until the sex act had been completed. This would lead me to believe that the body regards sex and the procreation of life as the most vital function of the human body and all else is secondary.

You may not agree with me but I repeat that what I have told you is the absolute truth and it did not take place on just one or two occasions but on many occasions throughout my lifetime. Therefore, for any doctor or individual to suggest that you avoid sex when you are suffering from arthritis or some other pain is, in my opinion, very bad advice. I would say to enjoy sex as much as possible or at least as much as your body demands.

CHAPTER 19

ASPIRIN

The medical profession leans heavily on aspirin, as does the Arthritis Foundation . . . both claiming it is still the number one drug in the treatment of arthritis.

What they really mean to say is that the pain-dulling qualitites of aspirin are the best means of combatting arthritis that they have at their disposal. They also probably mean that it does less damage than any other drug that they can prescribe.

When they say that aspirin is their best tool in the treatment of arthritis, I sincerely believe that they mean what they say and they are trying to do the arthritis sufferer a favor. Yes, I'm completely serious about this. After all, there are tens of thousands of other drugs on the market, most of which are more expensive and more deadly.

Now, if a doctor wants to keep on good terms with the American Medical Association, he will just have to go along with this accepted principle of prescribing aspirin for arthritis. Furthermore, if he doesn't want to harm his patients with the other drugs, prescribing aspirin is the best and kindest act he can perform. In this manner he keeps his nose clean and stays in tune with the American Medical Association and the

Arthritis Foundation.

However, let's examine the records to see if aspirin is as harmless as we are led to believe.

Here is what Dr. Paul Dudley White has to say in his work on heart disease, "Aspirin used over a long period of time may depress the production rate of the body's immune system and thus undermine the body's own healing powers."

The Journal of the American Medical Association of 1911 tells us that even small doses of aspirin can cause cardiac weakness with excessive pulse rate, edematous swelling of the mucous membrane, irregular pulse and occasionally albuminaria.

It has long been known that even one or two aspirin tablets can cause internal haemorrhages, as well as delerium and a state of incoherency, restlessness and confusion. Aspirin has been proven to be a vitamin antagonist, being especially antagonistic to Vitamin C, and will destroy massive quantities of Vitamin C if they are in the body. This was dealt with in an article in the Nutritional Review, 13, 46, 1955.

Here we have a report from the fifth World Congress of Gastroenterology held in Mexico City, as told in a newspaper from Long Beach, California, dated October 17, 1974:

"Heavy aspirin users may find themselves with some bigger headaches than the ones they're trying to cure: gastric ulcers, bleeding ulcers, ulcerative colitis and other severe intestinal problems.

"That's the consensus of some of the world's top specialists on stomach and intestinal ailments attending the fifth World Congress of Gastroenterology.

"Dr. Morton I. Grossman of UCLA said in an interview that one-third of those suffering from gastric ulcers are chronic, heavy aspirin users.

"He said some victims take huge quantities of aspirin to

control arthritis but the majority 'are just chronic aspirin users. They take it for headaches and often they can't tell you why.'

"Dr. Atanas Maleev, deputy minister of public health and director of the Academy of Medicine in Bulgaria, said: 'We have observed that 50 per cent of the bleeding ulcers, ulcerative colitis and serious lesions in the intestines seem to be directly related to patients who abuse the use of aspirin.' "

According to a copy of the Medical Letter, dated December 20, 1974, here is another drug for the treatment of arthritis which is classed as being better than aspirin:

"Ibuprofen (Motrin-Upjohn) is a new analgesic drug with anti-inflammatory activity, approved for use in rheumatoid arthritis and osteoarthritis. It is the first of several new nonsteroid antiarthritic drugs, available for several years in Canada and Europe, to be approved for use in the United States by the Food and Drug Administration. The manufacturer claims that ibuprofen is as effective as aspirin for treatment of arthritis, with fewer adverse effects.

"CLINICAL STUDIES — The effectiveness of ibuprofen for treatment of arthritis is dose related. The usual dosage suggested by the American manufacturer is 900 to 1600 mg daily, with a maximum of 2400 mg per day. In daily doses of less than 1600 mg, ibuprofen apparently does not have an anti-inflammatory effect in man, although even low doses have an analgesic effect; single doses of 300 and 900 mg of ibuprofen were similar in effectiveness to 900 mg of aspirin in relieving the pain of episiotomy (S. S. Bloomfield et al., Clin. Pharmacol. Ther., 15:565, June 1974). In short-term clinical trials in patients with arthritis, however, as much as 1200 mg of ibuprofen per day in divided doses was only intermediate in effectiveness between placebo and 3600 to 4000 mg of aspirin (E. F. Davies and G. S. Avery, Drugs, 2:416, 1971); in

117

one study, 900 mg of ibuprofen daily was no more effective than a placebo (P. L. Boardman et al., Ann. Rheum. Dis., 26:560, 1967). In a double-blind cross-over trial, 1200 mg of ibuprofen per day was less effective than 75 mg of indomethacin (Indocin) in the short-term treatment of osteoarthrosis of the hips (B. D. Owen-Smith and H. C. Burry, Rheumatol. Phys. Med., 11:281, 1972).

"Medical Letter consultants report that ibuprofen has anti-inflammatory effects at about 1600 to 2400 mg per day, and that in this dosage range ibuprofen appears to be as effective as usual doses of aspirin for the treatment of rheumatoid arthritis or osteoarthritis. Most of the experience with the drug has, however, been with a dosage of 1200 mg per day or less and the safety of higher dosages, especially with long-term use, is not well established.

"ADVERSE EFFECTS — The manufacturer claims that ibuprofen causes less gastrointestinal toxicity than aspirin. In one study, five days of treatment with ibuprofen, 800 to 1800 mg per day, causes less occult bleeding than 4800 mg of aspirin daily (M. Thompson and M. Anderson, Rheumatol. Phys. Med., Suppl:104, 1970). Gastrointestinal disturbances have, however, been reported with ibuprofen; the manufacturer estimates the incidence at four to 15 per cent. One Medical Letter consultant reports that some patients taking 1800 to 2400 mg of ibuprofen daily have developed gastritis, gastric ulceration, and such lower bowel symptoms as distention and diarrhea. Whether the gastrointestinal toxicity of high doses of ibuprofen taken over a long period of time will equal or exceed that of aspirin remains to be seen."

According to Bruce's Materia Medica, salicylic acid (commonly called aspirin) is rapidly absorbed and circulates as sodium salicylate and "a moderate dose causes a more rapid heart beat, a rise in blood pressure, flushing and warmth of the surface, perspiration, dullness in the head, tinnitus [ringing in the ears], deafness, impairment of vision and possibly slight fall in temperature. Larger doses may cause deliriums, especially with hallucinations; respiration is disturbed; the heart is slowed and weakened; the vessels are relaxed and the blood pressure falls."

In J. I. Rodale's book, "The Best Health Articles from Prevention", we read:

"The press was recently shaken by the statement of Dr. James Roth, professor of gastroenterology at the University of Pennsylvania Graduate School of Medicine, warning that aspirin is dangerous in any form. . . .

"Dr. Roth's opinion is that 60 to 70 per cent of all people who take aspirin in almost any form will bleed internally in small amounts. Most will lose only a teaspoon or so of blood, but occasionally a patient taking aspirin will lose as much as 3 ounces internally without even knowing it and once in a while a really severe hemorrhage can occur."

From the same source we read:

"A blood problem created by aspirin was discussed in the British Medical Journal, May 7, 1960. Two doctors called attention to aspirin's anticoagulant powers and warned that persons whose blood is already slow to coagulate take a serious risk in using aspirin, for it lowers even more the amount of the element in the blood, prothrombin, largely responsible for coagulation.

"Work on aspirin and its effect on the thyroid was reported in the Lancet (April 30, 1960). The observers found that, while there was no direct effect on the thyroid, salicylates interfered with the production of a hormone that stimulates the thyroid's activity. The net effect is that thyroxin, the vital secretion of the thyroid gland, is diminished. In cases in which the thyroid is already

119

underactive, salicylates could be an extremely dangerous drug, especially if used over a long period of time."

From "Vitamins in Medicine," by Bicknell and Prescott:

"Huebner and Link have shown that dicumarol, which produces a hypoprothrombinaemia, can be degraded to salicylic acid. It has been shown that salicylic acid and aspirin can induce hypoprothrombinaemia, which can be prevented by vitamin K. The possible clinical significance of the prothrombinopenic action of salicylates and aspirin has been discussed by clinicians, who suggest the use of Vitamin K prophylactically to reduce the possibility of haemorrhage in patients receiving large doses of salicylates. Meyer and Howard suggest that the haemorrhagic manifestations of acute rheumatic fever may be due to heavy dosage with salicylates. Small gastric haemorrhages are known to occur after taking aspirin on an empty stomach. Shapiro has shown that approximately 1 mg. of menaphthone (menadione U.S.P.) will counteract the prothrombinopenic activity of 1 gram of acetylsalicylic acid (aspirin) in patients receiving prolonged therapy with this drug."

From an editorial that appeared in the Journal of the American Medical Association as long ago as October 5, 1940, regarding the use of aspirin:

"Many reports have appeared on the adverse effects which may follow its unwise use. These have included depression of the heart, habit formation, miscarriage in pregnancy, and idiosyncrasy (allergic reaction) causing such alarming symptoms as urticaria (hives), pruritis (itching), erythema (redness of skin) and generalized angioneurotic edema (swelling of the skin due to a blood vessel disorder) . . . even ulceration and gangrene have been attributed to its use."

The following is quoted from the Merck Index regarding

the medical use of aspirin:

"**Med. Use:** Analgesic, antipyretic, antirheumatic. Occasionally employed in gout for its uricosuric and analgesic effect. Dose: Oral 0.3 to 1 gram. *Human Toxicity:* Average doses but more commonly large doses may cause tinnitus, nausea, vomiting, diarrhea, G. I. bleeding. Large doses may, in addition, cause auditory impairment, vertigo, headache, hyperpnea, acidosis, fever, diaphoresis, thirst, blurring of vision, skin eruptions, tachycardia, restlessness, hallucinations, delirium, stupor, coma, convulsions, circulatory collapse, respiratory failure, death. Prolonged use of average or large doses may produce hypoprothrombinemia and hemorrhage. Rarely, secondary thrombo-cytopenic purpura has been reported. The large doses required in rheumatic fever may cause mild Cushing's syndrome or occult edema. Doses over 3 g. have resulted in renal damage. Single dose of 10 to 30 g. usually fatal. Idiosyncrasy uncommon but appears most often in asthmatics (symptoms: mild to severe, sometimes fatal allergic reactions)."

From News and World Report, August 4, 1975 we read:

"Present indications are that the FDA aspirin rules will be these:

*Do not take more than two standard-sized pills at a time, every three to four hours — nor more than 12 in a day — for headache, fever, arthritis or rheumatism pain.

*Do not take aspirin, even in the recommended dosages, more than 10 days in succession.

*Do not take it if suffering from stomach problems, asthma or bleeding problems.

*Stop taking aspirin at once if it causes dizziness, ringing in the ears or chest pain. These could be signs of a dangerous allergic reaction to the drug. . . .

"It is a synthetic compound — acetylsalicylic acid —

121

which is made from petrochemicals. That is the product used today."

Now that you have had this chance to review but a few minuscule pieces of the mass of evidence telling of the harm, the danger and the destructive effects of aspirin, would you be willing to accept the doctor's cliche, "Aspirin is the medical profession's best drug"?

CHAPTER 20

FASTING AS A TREATMENT FOR ARTHRITIS

At the outset I want to make it clear that I believe fasting to be one of the greatest therapeutic measures known to mankind. I think the experts on fasting call it, 'Physiological Rest.' They give it other names as well, but no matter what they call it or how they refer to it, it is still fasting. I do not like to refer to it as the "deprivation of food" because some authorities will take exception to this and say that you are not being deprived of food because your body has built up a store of fat and you will live on it if you get down to real hunger.

Let me explain that there are at least two kinds of fasting. One is a total fast wherein you partake of only water which the experts say must be distilled water at that, so that you do not ingest any of the organic or inorganic minerals which are usually found in water. The second type of fast is the one that is more often practised in Europe (in fact, they call it the European fast) wherein they use fruit and vegetable juices but no solid food.

In Germany there is one of the largest and best known fasting institutions in the world and from first hand information, I believe they have chalked up remarkable results with their means and method of fasting ... that is, using juices of various kinds but no solid food. I understand that they also use various broths or soups in the European fast.

Today the foremost proponent and exponent of the first system of fasting, that is the total fast, is Dr. Herbert M. Shelton, who operates Dr. Shelton's Health School in San Antonio, Texas. I understand that they have fasted more than 50,000 people there but, whether or not all of these people fasted their way back to health, I am not prepared to say. From the best information at my disposal I believe there are at least six fasting institutions based on the Shelton system in the United States at the present time, but there may be many more.

Here I would like to give my views concerning the total fast and the European fast. If I were fasting, I would make mine the total fast ... mainly because I feel that the effects of the physiological rest would not be accomplished if I drank fruit and vegetable juices, which no one can deny are still food. To me a fast is the abandonment of food for a given period. Therefore, if you are going to fast, I would recommend the total fast wherein you only partake of water.

From what I have seen and learned, I would say that there are very, very few people who would not benefit from a fast unless it's those starving people in various parts of the world. But I sincerely feel that most of the people in America would benefit materially by a fast. No, I am not suggesting that 100% of the people in America would benefit from a fast but I do think that the majority of them most certainly would — even those who are not overweight. The reason I say this is because I don't know of one person in America who eats a completely proper diet and if you do not eat properly, your body accumulates toxic substances of various kinds taken in with food and these should be eliminated. Well, the best way and perhaps in some cases the only way to eliminate them is through a fast.

It is claimed that there are two common conditions for which a fast would not be desirable or indicated . . . or maybe I should say, for which a fast is contra-indicated. The two conditions are diabetes and cancer and, basically, I am inclined to agree with this finding.

Fasting is no great complicated affair and I feel that anyone can fast from three to five days without any special supervision. Just do a bit of reading on the subject, use a bit of common sense and make sure you drink plenty of water.

In my opinion one need not use distilled water when fasting. In fact, I think you would get better results with plain, ordinary water. However, chlorinated or fluoridated water should be avoided like the plague. I would suggest that when you undertake a fast you get yourself some good spring water.

I would strongly urge anyone who wants to fast beyond five days to do so under proper supervision in one of the institutions throughout America. For myself, however, I think I could safely fast for ten or even twenty days without any special supervision. In fact, friends of mine have undergone ten to fourteen day fasts without any supervision . . . but with great benefits. However, you must know what you are doing.

To set the records straight, I went on one twenty-one day fast (under supervision) and there were no complications whatsoever. However, you can't depend on clear sailing during the frequent longer fasts where one may run into a crisis and where, without proper supervision, you may run into serious problems. So take my word for it . . . if you intend to fast for more than five days, go to an institution.

On many occasions through the past 20 years I have undergone a three day fast and on a few occasions I have undergone a five day fast. Actually I have benefitted from all of these short fasts and I think it is a mighty good idea to fast for two or three days every now and then — especially if you have some gastro-intestinal or other disturbances. I have also gone on many one day fasts — especially in my travels. While travelling I sometimes run into problems. But at home I try to eat and live right so that fasting is unnecessary. However, if I feel something is wrong, I just stop eating. I will not even accept a cup of tea of any kind.

Something I want to make very clear is that while I consider periodic short fasts to be beneficial — that is, one to five day fasts — a longer fast than that should not be repeated. I warn you, long fasts should not be repeated.

Now I am basing my opinion upon actual cases and observation, where people have undergone a thirty day fast or longer and then a little while later, even a year or two later, they underwent another thirty day fast. In these cases the fasting turned out to be harmful . . . not just without benefit, but harmful.

I strongly warn all my readers that if you undergo one long fast make sure that you will never have to undergo another long fast because the second fast may do serious harm or be your undoing.

If, for example, you are suffering from some condition and you decide to undergo a fast at one of the institutions, where you might fast ten, twenty or thirty days — which is not unusual — when you have finished that fast, resolve there and then that you will live so that there will be no necessity for another such fast as long as you live.

I do know people of the hygienic group, who undergo annual fasts of ten, fourteen or more days but none of them are really healthy in my estimation. In most cases they undergo these fasts to compensate for their gluttony or dietary errors. One friend of mine, a famous medical specialist whom I introduced to fasting, found fasting so beneficial that he made an annual fetish of it . . . until it killed him.

Here I would like to quote from a letter from the director at Dr. Shelton's Health School in San Antonio, Texas, dated March 31, 1975:

"100 per cent of arthritics that come to the Health School improve or completely recover their health. Whether or not they improve or recover completely depends on the amount of pathologic deterioration which has taken place. Sometimes for complete recovery, more than one fast is required. Most joints that were immovable before the fast are more mobile after the fast and with each succeeding fast there is greater and greater mobility. To continue to improve after one fast one must carry out the Hygienic way of life 100 per cent.

"I have been reading your articles on fasting with interest and I think that seeing people who have not carried out the Hygienic way of life after the fast has distorted your view of multiple fasting. I have had spectacular recoveries of health by having the invalid take more than one long fast, whereas he would not have achieved these results had he not taken another fast.

"You have seen people return from the Health School weak and enervated. Rather than wait out that period of weakness and continue in their Hygienic program, they begin searching for short-cuts and miracle cures, hence they do not ever regain their strength and health as they do not continue the Hygienic program. It is unfortunate that there is so little understanding of Hygiene and fasting even among those who profess to be our friends.

"Many times, instead of reconsulting a Hygienic practitioner, these invalids will seek the guidance of a

Naturopath or a health food store salesman and consequently are steered wrongly in their way of life and given false ideas.

"Dr. Shelton joins me in sending you our kindest regards."

There is one other thing about fasting that I would like to point out at this time and that is that one should never undergo a long fast needlessly. Three of my acquaintances through the years underwent long fasts without need. That is, they just felt that they would like to try it and perhaps benefit themselves or lose some weight . . . but they all suffered seriously. In some instances people never totally recover their health.

My warning, after taking all available opinions into consideration, is still, "Don't fast needlessly or frivolously and don't go on a long fast more than once."

Let's say you are suffering from arthritis and come to me for advice. You have been to doctors, taken drugs and had all of their treatments, with no results or even a worsening of the condition. You are desperate and you say to me, "Please help me!"

It is my sincere conviction that the best method to bring arthritis under control is a fast followed by a 100% raw food diet. If you could afford it I would advise you to go to a good fasting institution and place yourself in their competent care. If you could not afford it, I would suggest that you buy two or three books on fasting (Carrington is one of the best), study them and then follow their teachings.

For those who are capable and have the will power, I would strongly recommend a short fast, followed by a totally raw food diet of vegetables, grains, fruits and nuts. There is no method on earth to compare with this treatment. Best of all, you can do it all by yourself . . . no supervision or institutionalizing is required.

128

CHAPTER 21

MINERAL BATHS, SPAS AND CLIMATIC CHANGES

It is quite within the realm of possibility that mineral baths, spas and climatic changes may have their place in the treatment of arthritis because I have met many people who claimed they were helped and some who claimed they were cured by one or all of these methods.

Yes, I will concede that it could be that these methods do have their place in the healing of arthritis . . . especially if you would seek to avoid making changes in your living and dietary habits. In my estimation, judging from years of observation, there appears to be little danger of harm from these means and methods, so if you are suffering you might as well try whatever you can. Seeking help from one of these sources is as logical as any other devious course that you may care to pursue. When you are suffering, you are entitled to seek relief.

I have a relative who began to have arthritic pain in his early forties. He was treated by medical doctors, chiropractors, osteopaths and herbal healers . . . all without relief. He even took the gold cure; then he bounced down to Mt. Clements in Michigan for the mineral springs treatment; then he went to California for the mineral mud treatment and then he went on to Arizona to the desert to lie in the sun. Oh, yes, he went down into a mine for a cure, too. He sat in this damp, dreary, dark mine for many hours each day and for many days. From all of these he claimed that he did get some relief. Well, he is still alive today — in his late 80's — although he has not changed his ways one bit. He claims that the pain has mainly subsided, although he still has some pain and some crippling. I know all about his diet and I state that he eats the ideal arthritic's diet . . . delicious, rich and almost entirely cooked food.

It is obvious that arthritis is a crippler and a pain-giver but it is not an out-and-out killer. Arthritis, as a rule, will stick with you as long as you live . . . that is, if you refuse to change your diet and your way of living. However, those who are willing to change their ways can have the condition alleviated and even arrested.

I felt that the radon mine treatment should at least be given mention and I am quoting from the literature that I received from John T. Lewis, President of the Free Enterprise Uranium-Radon Mine, written by Harold R. Tregilgas, M.D., F.A.C.S., in collaboration on research with Wade V. Lewis, B.S., Geologist.

"For 10 years the Free Enterprise Uranium-Radon Mine at Boulder, Montana, has been in continuous operation. Initially it was the first commercial uranium ore producer of Montana. It is now operated as a means of affording relief to those afflicted with arthritis, bursitis, sinusitis, neuritis, asthma, and other chronic, painful conditions which the medical profession is often unable to clear up with regular treatment.

"As a medical doctor, my conclusions regarding benefits accruing to the mine visitor are based on personal observation and experience, as well as upon reports from other sources. In

130

1959, I developed a painful stiffness and swelling in both hands, right arm, shoulders, and neck. This condition increased in severity, making it difficult to continue surgery.

"I visited the Free Enterprise Mine, taking, over a 10-day period, about 30 hours of exposure to radon and its transmuted solid elements. Within weeks I experienced elimination of pain, stiffness and swelling of body members. I have had no signs or symptoms of arthritis since, and have taken no aspirin for pain for the past two years.

"Since visiting the Free Enterprise Radon Mine I have sent many cases there, a high percentage of which responded favorably to the treatment.

"Results attained at the Free Enterprise Mine, especially for rheumatoid arthritis, are not without precedent. In 1934, the beneficial effect of radon, present in more meager amounts in springs and spas, was discussed by Francis J. Scully, M.D., in a bulletin entitled 'The Role of Radioactivity of Natural Spring Waters as a Therapeutic Agent,' reprinted from the *Journal* of the Arkansas Medical Society, Vol. XXX, March, 1934, pp. 206-214. Dr. Scully emphasizes that radon can be employed for a long period of time without any adverse after-effects and states that arthritis in all forms benefits from this type of treatment. . . .

"A parallel to the Free Enterprise Radon Mine operation is found at Bad Gastein, Austria, where a 1,500 meter adit affords a copious amount of radon gas. German pamphlets reporting on European arthritics show clinical evaluations virtually identical to observations at the Montana radon mine.

"The Bad Gastein mine is described in the *Journal* of the American Medical Association, June 30, 1956, Vol. 161, No. 9, p. 917, under *Medical Literature Abstracts,* in an article entitled 'Combined Treatment by Radium Emanation and Hyperthermy of Bad Gastein,' by Dr. Otto Henn. The *Journal* article, in referring to radon gas, concludes:

" 'It exerts an influence on the autonomic nervous system, improves the circulatory state, and causes removal of waste from the organism and an activation of hormone producing organs, particularly of the pituitary-adrenal system. Indications and contraindications for this type of treatment are apparently the same as those for corticotropin (ACTH) and cortisone therapy.' . . .

"Evidently two principal environmental factors in nature account for the physical improvements now claimed by those thousands who have visited Free Enterprise Mine: (1) radon therapy, the utilization of radon's transmuted elements, producing mild but effective internal radiation reaching the blood stream, the body cells, and the endocrine gland system; (2) ionization, a product of radon's radiation, reported as stimulating defense cells of the body, inducing better utilization of oxygen.

"A recent paper entitled 'Medical Hydrology,' by Igho Hart Kornbleuh, M.D. and Paul K. Kuroda, Ph.D., states:

" 'Studies of the biologic influence of unipolarly ionized air show some striking similarities to the effects of radium emanation (radon). The results so far achieved indicate that inhalation of this gas or of ionized air is by far most effective. . . . Clinical evaluations have established the following effects of radon: A pain controlling quality, stimulation of the inner secretory glands, increased diuresis and excretion of uric acid as its most conspicuous properties.

" 'It appears that radon in carefully controlled quantities exerts a rather specific eubiotic influence without any undesirable aftereffects.' . . .

"According to an article entitled 'Ions Can Do Strange Things to You,' written by Robert O'Brien and appearing in the *Reader's Digest* of October, 1960, experiments are going forward at Northeastern Hospital in Philadelphia, using artificially developed ionization for post surgical pain and particularly for severe burn cases. The article states:

" 'Negative ions in the blood stream accelerate delivery of oxygen to our cell and tissues. . . . Researchers also believe that negative ions may stimulate the reticulo-endothelial system, a group of defense cells which marshal our resistance to disease.' "

"Other sources claim that the internal radiation acquired at the Free Enterprise Mine stimulates the boss pituitary gland in its production of ACTH, the latter acting upon the adrenal cortex in its production of hydrocortisone, the body pain killer. . . .

"In October, 1961, an International Conference on Ionization was held at the Franklin Institute, Philadelphia, sponsored by the American Institute of Medical Climatology. Medical doctors, as well as those from other professions, attended from France, Germany, Sweden, Denmark, Russia, and the United States. Proceedings of this meeting emphasized the importance of ionization for body well-being.

"It is evident that physical benefits observed at the Free Enterprise Radon Mine are due to induced body chemical changes, increased body hormone production, and are certainly not of psychosomatic origin, except to the extent normally anticipated by any kind of therapy.

"The subject of radon gas, its transmuted elements and attending ionization, certainly merits further research, under careful medical supervision. Such studies should be very rewarding and worthwhile."

The following is a paragraph from a leaflet addressed, "To All Free Enterprise Mine Visitors":

"Those claiming the most relief and benefits after visiting the Free Enterprise Uranium-Radon Mine have taken a series of 12 to 32 one-hour visits as a rule, two visits each day — one in the morning and one in the afternoon. Those visitors taking less hours' exposure usually write in and say, 'I have received benefits but feel that I would have benefited much more had I visited longer.' "

From a personal letter I received from John T. Lewis, President of Free Enterprise Uranium-Radon Mine, I quote the following:

"We appreciate your good ethics as a journalist in coming to us for the facts, and will be happy to show you the mine, should you ever decide to visit out here."

I feel that this organization is on the up-and-up. They are not trying to make a killing and they are not holding anyone for ransom. Their rates appear to be reasonable . . . in fact, low as compared to most other means and methods of treatment offered.

My conclusion concerning the Free Enterprise Uranium-Radon Mine is that it bears investigation or trial for sufferers who, for various reasons, cannot or will not follow a proper raw food diet as I advocate. The raw food diet is without a doubt the most effective method on earth. Personally — and I state this clearly, unmistakably and with great emphasis — I have a built-in fear of any form of radiation, apart from that distributed by the sun and the atmosphere.

Just how radioactive substances can be of help to arthritic sufferers is beyond my comprehension. However, from the evidence that I have read, it would appear that a great number of people have been helped at least temporarily by a visit to the uranium-radon mine. Perhaps radiation from minimal natural source emanation is less harmful . . . but I could never, under any circumstances, accept the fact that radiation could ever genuinely benefit the body.

However, I feel it is my duty to clearly point out that

radiation in various forms is often beneficial or at least harmless in the early stages of exposure . . . but what happens 5, 10 or 20 years later may tell an entirely different story. You wouldn't be wise if you traded your arthritis of today for a bit of relief by radium exposure and then wound up with a form of non-curable cancer in 5, 10 or 20 years.

Cancer is usually the result in the medical use of radiation. Therefore, my conclusion about radium or kindred substance mines and treatment is that you'd best leave them alone. To me it sounds like "relief today . . . cancer later."

I feel that sustained or repeated radium exposure ultimately kills everything it touches!

Through the years I have known people who tried every known avenue. Even if they had to travel 5,000 miles, it made no difference . . . they went. If they had to immerse themselves in hot, almost boiling water or mud, they did it. Then there are thousands who seek the warmer, drier climates and claim they get relief. Some even claim they are cured as long as they remain there. To me, it all adds up to one thing . . . they will do anything on earth except what they ought to do, which is live according to the law of nature.

CHAPTER 22

COD LIVER OIL AND ARTHRITIS

Vitamin D and cod liver oil have always been mentioned as though they were synonymous terms because of the high Vitamin D content of the oil.

Various authors and individuals try to make it appear that cod liver oil is the great benefactor of the arthritis sufferer, so I have taken the time and the trouble to thoroughly investigate the merits of the cod liver oil treatment of arthritis. I ask you to weigh the evidence.

Even though cod liver oil has been used for well over 100 years, I still maintain that it does not belong in the human diet. It is quite all right to have the oil of the cod as found when eating cod fish but I think that separating the oil from the liver of the cod by various processes — including allowing the liver to rot to extract the oil as a food supplement — and then ingesting that oil is totally wrong. This practice can do nothing but bring ultimate harm to those who follow it.

My reply to those who claim that they have had beneficial results from the use of cod liver oil is, "It is not food for man nor beast and can never bring any good to anyone. The benefits that you derived were due to the other changes that you made in your diet and living habits and not from the cod liver oil."

As part of the cod liver oil treatment, fresh squeezed orange juice or milk is used with the cod liver oil. Where the patient was sensitive to orange juice, then milk was given in its place.

One of the musts or positive requisites for those on the cod liver oil treatment was the complete elimination of all soft drinks, candy, cake, ice-cream or any food made with white sugar. It also recommended giving up coffee but they made an allowance for those who considered the lack of coffee a hardship and coffee was permitted at least 15 minutes before breakfast, provided water was given first.

I would like to make the challenging statement that if the arthritic sufferer did nothing but give up coffee, soft drinks, candy, cake, ice cream or any food made with white sugar for a thirty day period, the arthritic condition would undoubtedly improve noticeably . . . and this could be accomplished without the use of the horrendous, vile tasting, ill-smelling, despicable and harmful cod liver oil. In fact, I would emphatically state that the improvement would be much greater if the cod liver oil were omitted.

I do believe though that the use of cod liver oil as a medicine has worked by disguising or altering the existing symptoms — be it symptoms of rickets, arthritis or any other disease — but I suggest that it is only trading one condition or disease for another. I think cod liver oil causes or contributes to more serious conditions. My advice to those who are seeking health is not to seek to alter the existing disease or condition but to correct it.

Professor Henrik Dam of Copenhagen and his co-workers administered large quantities of cod liver oil to experimental animals, which resulted in severe disorders of the skin and other organs if the diet of these animals was lacking in Vitamin E. It was discovered that when Vitamin E or tocopherols were added in sufficient amounts all signs of illness disappeared in a rather short time.

The Danish investigators made another discovery. When examining the animal bodies, they found deposits of dark colored peroxides of fatty acids in the arteries in various parts of the animal bodies if there was not sufficient Vitamin E in the diet. This indicates in the most definite terms possible that if you insist upon taking cod liver oil . . . be sure that you are also getting adequate quantities of Vitamin E.

Cod liver oil has to be purified and put through various processes before anyone can put his nose even close to it. Remember, most of the oil comes from the rotting livers of cod fish, so all cod liver oil is rancid or was rancid . . . but the rancidity has been disguised by some devious chemical means. So how could it be a healthful product?

I quote from Bicknell and Prescott's book, "The Vitamins In Medicine":

"Rancid Fats: Their Destruction of Vitamin E and their Relation to Muscular Dystrophy. Rancid fats rapidly destroy vitamin E by oxidation. This destruction is most liable to occur when vitamin E is in the form of the synthetic vitamin or concentrated preparations, since then it is no longer protected against oxidation by the anti-oxidants found associated with it in such natural sources as whole wheat germ."

It is important that you understand that rancid fats rapidly destroy Vitamin E by oxidation, as was proven by Bicknell and Prescott.

I have a reference here concerning an experiment conducted by a researcher by the name of Adamstone. His work suggests that cod liver oil causes intestinal sarcoma in

139

fowl that are deficient in Vitamin E . . . and practically every person in America is deficient in Vitamin E because of all the refined foods eaten today.

My feeling is, if you are willing to take the risk of changing arthritis into cancer, then and then only, continue using gobs of cod liver oil as recommended by some writers.

It is my contention, supported by documented research data, that an over-abundance of Vitamin D can cause many serious conditions and cod liver oil does supply tremendous quantities of Vitamin D to the body. Those writers who recommend that large doses of cod liver oil be taken regularly must be unmindful of the fact that this means ingesting enormous doses of Vitamin D. Again, I repeat, taking large doses of cod liver oil is a seriously dangerous practice and I suggest that we let those who recommend it take it themselves!

Some conditions that overdoses of cod liver oil will cause are rough skin, weight loss, gastrointestinal disorders, diarrhea and calcium deposits in various parts of the body, such as in the large blood vessels, in the heart and the kidneys. It contributes to nephritis and uremic symptoms. Uremic symptoms are due to toxicosis from protein disintegration.

If rats kept on a certain standard diet well suited for breeding purposes receive a larger dose of cod liver oil daily, they become ill. If guinea pigs on a scurvy-producing diet are protected against it by supplementing fruit juices, additions of cod liver oil remove the antiscorbutic action of the fruit juices.

Furthermore, hypervitaminosis D (which means an overdose of Vitamin D) is an action upon the fat metabolism resulting in emaciation, lipoid infiltration of the liver, arterial wall and endocrine glands. In dealing with test animals it was found that in high dosage it causes calcium deposits, cachexia and death of the test animals. In this respect'it is a poison for man as well.

The above information is researched from the work of some of the best authorities in the world on the toxicity and benefits of Vitamin D, so I beg you not to ignore these warnings. Here I would like to name a few of the research authorities: Stepp, Kuhnau, Schroeder, Bicknell, Prescott, Holtz, Von Brand, De Moles, Harris, Moore, Juswitz, Banberger, Degkwitz, Pfannfstiel, Kreitmair and Moll.

Now don't run off with the idea that if you take large doses of Vitamin D the body can slough it off and get rid of it as it wants because this is not true. In an experiment conducted with feeding cows large doses of Vitamin D, it was found that only 25% of the huge doses of Vitamin D that were fed were eliminated with the feces and no Vitamin D at all was found in the urine. Somehow the body builds up or stores or hides the Vitamin D and that is obviously what does the harm. Think about this before you ever embark on the cod liver oil treatment for arthritis. Otherwise, I suggest that you will be going from the frying pan into the fire.

However, Dr. Eddy in The Avitaminoses, states, "It is apparent that the danger of overdosage is remote when the usual preparations of vitamin D are used. The early symptoms of vitamin D 'poisoning,' as it is called, are: nausea, loss of appetite, vomiting, cramps, diarrhea, tingling in the fingers and toes, dizziness and so forth. Of course, these are symptoms of many other disorders, too. When you get too much vitamin D, your body does not use calcium properly any longer and this is what causes the complaints. In some way not understood by physiologists, vitamin D controls calcium and phosphorus in your body. If there is not enough vitamin D, this machinery will go awry. If there is too much, it will go wrong in a different way."

Granted, cod liver oil does help bowel movements and practically eliminates constipation, but there is a very, very good reason for this . . . it causes diarrhea to a lesser or greater degree. The body recognizes that it is harmful and tries to get rid of it as quickly as possible and thus you have diarrhea or the good bowel movements. Remember, these bowel movements are attained at a very high price as far as your health is concerned because many good and essential nutrients go out with the cod liver oil in the bowel movement.

When cod liver oil is used in large quantities, it can be a causative factor in muscular dystrophy, as the following quote from "The Vitamins In Medicine" proves:

"When Goettsch and Pappenheimer first reported nutritional muscular dystrophy, they did not consider a deficiency of vitamin E was the cause because wheat germ oil supplements failed to prevent the dystrophy. It now can be seen that this was because their diet contained so much cod liver oil and lard that the vitamin taken in the wheat germ oil was destroyed during digestion in the stomach."

Now I would like to make one further statement about this cod liver oil affair. I have talked to many people who take cod liver oil and in not one single instance did I find an individual who was healthy. They all had one, two or many conditions from which they were suffering. Of course, the reason is obvious . . . if they are taking cod liver oil, they already had trouble and, as long as they take it, they will have greater trouble.

CHAPTER 23

CIDER VINEGAR AND HONEY

No doubt you have heard of Dr. D. C. Jarvis and his famous book, "Folk Medicine."

I read this book when it first came off the press many years ago because I had had problems in my legs, my arms and, especially, my elbows. The remedy that he suggested — namely, cider vinegar and honey — was so simple and actually pleasant to take that I felt I must give it a try.

I immediately bought a jug of apple cider vinegar and a four pound pail of honey and I went to work on them as he suggested. Incidentally, it was also claimed, I believe, that it would make you slimmer at the same time.

For months I faithfully indulged in this remedy but I noticed no change in my condition, so I discontinued taking the concoction.

Now just about the time I discontinued Dr. Jarvis's remedy of cider vinegar and honey, I began to develop a keen interest in the topic of enzymes. I soon learned that enzymes were a vital factor in human nutrition ... something that the medical profession and the nutritional scientists had ignored or failed to notice. I discovered that without enzymes the food one eats can never be fully or properly metabolized.

I soon learned that only natural raw substances contain enzymes and that these enzymes are destroyed when temperatures exceed 140 degrees Fahrenheit. Well, I felt reasonably sure that the cider vinegar and honey that I was taking were both pasteurized, which meant that they had been heated above 140 degrees . . . so they would have little merit as a nutritive or a curative agent.

I went out to try to get unpasteurized apple cider vinegar and unpasteurized honey. An apiarist nearby agreed he would not pasteurize the honey and I could have it in its natural form, but I came up against a veritable stone wall when I tried to get unpasteurized apple cider vinegar.

I got in touch with practically every vinegar producing outfit in Canada but they all told me the same thing . . . they pasteurized all their vinegar. When I asked why, they said very simply, "If you don't pasteurize it, the apple cider vinegar will become darker in color and form 'mother,' which is a slimy mucus-like substance, and people just don't like having that in their vinegar. Once pasteurized it remains the same almost forever."

Please believe me, I searched from coast to coast before I finally found a small operator who had some unpasteurized apple cider vinegar . . . but since then the idea of natural, unpasteurized cider vinegar has grown and multiplied. Then I started to take the apple cider vinegar and honey again . . . but this time I made sure they were not pasteurized. However, I believe I was the first man in America to recognize the fact that the apple cider vinegar and the honey had to be in their natural, unpasteurized state if they were to function as Dr. Jarvis claimed.

Perhaps you wonder why honey is pasteurized. I think it is important that you know the reason. It is not for the consumer's benefit, it is purely a merchandising practice.

In the first place, 'pasteurized' is a miracle word to most people. It sounds pure and wholesome, without germs and bacteria. The truth is that the heat of the pasteurization process kills all the living organisms in the honey, thus making it little better than sugar. The only honey fit to eat is wholesome, natural, unprocessed and unpasteurized honey.

Now for the chief or real reason why honey is pasteurized. If stored in a container which is not tightly closed, unpasteurized honey, being hygroscopic, draws moisture from the air. This added moisture will cause fermentation and the honey will bubble up and expand tremendously and force its way out of the container. Then the grocer has a real mess to clean up because it flows down the shelves and all over. One such occurrence in a warehouse or supermarket and raw unpasteurized honey is 'verboten' for now and evermore.

You see, the supermarkets are not in the least concerned about the nutritive or health-contributing qualities of the honey . . . they just don't want a nasty mess or financial losses. So now you know why it is hard to get unpasteurized honey.

I'll tell you something else. Most honey that is supposed to be unpasteurized is really pasteurized. How do I know? I took the time and trouble to test it out by actually contacting many honey producers. I found out that while some did not actually put the honey through the pasteurization process as such, they heated the honey to the point of pasteurization or higher.

You just can't trust anyone, it seems, but at least you now know the truth. Test it out for yourself and you'll learn that I do know whereof I speak.

Again the months rolled by and I felt that I had had enough apple cider vinegar and honey, so I stopped taking it . . . after all, it was a bit of a bother. Then a few weeks later one of my knees buckled under me when I was descending the stairs in my home and I almost catapulted down. Suddenly the rude awakening struck . . . the apple cider vinegar and honey had worked. Also, I realized that after taking the remedy my elbows hadn't been as sensitive to knocks any more either.

Immediately I went back on the cider vinegar and honey regimen and I continued taking it until I switched to a mainly raw food diet, which I still continue today.

Just taking this apple cider vinegar and honey as a cure-all for arthritis did seem a bit far-fetched to me, I knew there were no magic potions, foods, miracle drugs or miracle cures, which I am sure any man with normal intelligence has learned although you wouldn't think so by the way everyone goes on searching for such cures. Then I began to ask myself questions as to why the apple cider vinegar and honey mixture was so effective.

In Jarvis's day there was no pasteurization of honey or apple cider vinegar, so they were probably two of the few raw substances that an individual ingested which contained their full allotment of enzymes intact. And if he took this mixture three or four times a day he would be getting a fairly decent amount of at least two raw food products. This is the only logical way I could figure it out and I feel sure I was basically right. Of course with this came the enlightenment that raw food is excellent food and one needs more of it . . . and from then on my nutritional awakening began to take place.

In case you have any doubts as to the effectiveness of Dr. Jarvis's cider vinegar and honey remedy in the treatment of arthritis, let me suggest that it can do you no harm and it invariably brings benefit to arthritis sufferers. It has been used successfully for over 50 years and it certainly is worth a try . . . but, remember, it doesn't work overnight. Allow two months before expecting any marked improvement.

Prior to the advent of this book by Dr. D. C. Jarvis, there was a smaller book entitled "Apple Cider Vinegar," written by Cyril Scott, the famous musician, and published in Britain. This little book, which is only a little bigger than a pamphlet, has sold hundreds of thousands, if not millions of copies in the English speaking world. When I read this book carefully I found that it was based on the information presented to the author, Cyril Scott, many years before by Dr. D. C. Jarvis. Then, after Jarvis saw the tremendous number of books that Cyril Scott had sold, he decided to publish his own book and he withdrew his permission for Cyril Scott to use his material.

What I am trying to tell you is that the knowledge that Dr. Jarvis passed on to Cyril Scott about the value of cider vinegar and honey in the treatment of arthritis and other pains has been a widely used remedy and no doubt through the years millions of people have been helped by it.

Now at this time, in case you think Dr. Jarvis was some kind of nut or quack, let me tell you that Dr. Jarvis was born in 1881, was a graduate of the University of Vermont Medical School and started practising medicine in Vermont in 1909. He was Editor of the Medical World and was a member of the Academy of Ophthalmology and Otolaryngology, the American Medical Association and other leading medical societies. His interest in the folk medicine of Vermont began soon after the start of his medical practice and he pursued his study of it for a lifetime.

Of course, Dr. Jarvis's book was a best seller. I don't know how many editions were printed but from the best information I have there are more than twenty editions in the hard back, apart from the paper back editions. It was first published in 1958.

Lest you laugh at the effectiveness of this simple folk remedy, I advise you to try it before you knock it! I have recommended the cider vinegar and honey treatment to hundreds of people and I have never known anyone to come back and say it didn't work. It did work, it does work and it will work.

Now I felt that the apple cider vinegar and honey concoction was good but not good enough for all of these heavy cooked-food eaters who were suffering from arthritis. I felt something better had to be done, so I dreamed up the idea of adding a teaspoonful of untreated alfalfa herb or powder to each glass of the mixture. The reason I added the alfalfa is because I consider alfalfa to be a splendid food and an extremely nutritive plant. I rank it among the best foods or grasses to be found in nature. It contains the widest list of elements found in any grass and it is capable of correcting many nutritional deficiencies that exist in the animal body.

Here is the actual formula as I used it, based upon Dr. Jarvis's apple cider vinegar and honey. Get one quart of unpasteurized apple cider vinegar and one four pound pail of unpasteurized honey (buckwheat, clover or whatever) but be positive that they are both unpasteurized . . . that is, not heated above 140 degrees. Pour the jug of vinegar into a bowl and stir in as much honey as the vinegar will absorb, stirring or mixing until it becomes a syrup. Put the mixture into a large bottle or container and keep it in the refrigerator. Then every day or better still, two or three times a day, take out a tablespoonful or two or three of the mixture and put it into a glass. Fill the glass with water, add one heaping teaspoonful of alfalfa powder, stir like 'crazy' and then drink. I used to drink this twice a day and sometimes three times a day.

Don't let anyone tell you that vinegar will dry up your

blood or any of that nonsense. If you take regular doses of strictly unpasteurized apple cider vinegar, unpasteurized honey and naturally dried alfalfa herb, that has been chopped or ground, you will probably be doing as much, in fact, more to help yourself back to health and rid yourself of arthritis than you could by following any known medical or surgical treatment. Furthermore, a month of treatment won't cost you more than a dollar or two and there will be no side-effects as is the case with drugs. Can an arthritis sufferer do more for himself?

Back a few years ago I sat in my office and watched a crippled, grey haired lady get out of a car with the aid of a pair of crutches. Then she hobbled into my business premises.

In those days, apart from my budding publishing business, I also had a natural food establishment. It was mainly a mail order business but we also served people who came to the door.

After a few minutes I decided to go out and see just what the score was. I sort of stood in the background for a while as she ordered a gallon of unpasteurized apple cider vinegar, which was the only kind we sold, a pail of unpasteurized honey and a package of alfalfa herb.

Just before she paid for her purchases I walked over to her and casually asked, "Have you ever used this stuff before?"

She answered, "Oh, yes, I have been using it for over a year."

Then, wearing my nastiest face, I said to her, "It hasn't done you much good, has it?"

She snapped back in a very sharp tone of voice, "That's what you think!"

She didn't know who I was and I didn't know who she was, but I said, "Please, forgive me, I shouldn't have spoken to you that way. But you told me you have been using this supposedly curative preparation for more than a year, yet you are using crutches."

Still in a rather icy voice, she replied, "But you didn't see me before I started taking it!"

I often use this form of inquisition to see what kind of reaction it will bring forth, so I went on in a rather reconciliatory tone, "Please, tell me more. I am genuinely interested and please be assured that I didn't mean to offend you. It is just that I have long known that this remedy is effectual and I was rather disappointed to see you hobbling in on those crutches."

"Let me tell you this," she said, "I was in a wheel chair for more than five years and the doctors told me that I would never walk again. In response to my pleas for help, the best they could offer me were aspirin and cortisone. I took both until I began to get some very serious side-effects. I decided to chuck the whole works and accept the fact that the doctors are stumbling along and don't know what they are doing. Then someone told me about this cider vinegar, honey and alfalfa concoction. I tried it and I have taken it ever since . . . and I will take it as long as I live."

"May I ask how old you are?" I queried.

"I am 79 years of age," she said.

Then I pushed the question forward, "Have you ever thought of going on a raw food diet?"

She said, "I have no intention of changing my ways. I have found that this concoction has helped me. I have been improving with each succeeding day and I feel certain that within the next year I will be able to discard the crutches, too."

"How often do you take this guck," I asked her.

"Twice a day," she replied.

"Just how do you mix it?" I then asked.

"A teaspoonful of honey, a tablespoonful of vinegar and then I fill the glass with water and stir in as much alfalfa as I can get on a teaspoon," she said.

I asked, "Why don't you try it three times a day?"

"I just don't want to overdo a good thing," she said. "Twice a day is working for me and I'm not changing."

I swear this story that I have related is absolutely true and you can take it for what it is worth. As I mentioned before, I feel that the reason this concoction works so well is because it is probably the most raw food and the best variety of raw food that these sufferers ever consume. This is one way of getting good wholesome natural food into their systems . . . food that has not been heat-treated or pasteurized.

After more than fifteen years of experience with this 'guck,' as I call it, I say unhesitatingly, that it will improve the condition of any sufferer of any form of arthritis. I advise anyone amd everyone who is suffering from arthritis to try this concoction of unpasteurized honey, apple cider vinegar and alfalfa. I say it works . . . no, not as well as a proper raw food diet, but it does work and it is quite effective . . . in fact, more effective than most people can possibly believe.

CHAPTER 24

VARIOUS TREATMENTS FOR ARTHRITIS

Paracelsus, one of the great men in healing, said:

"Wherever nature produces pain there she accumulates harmful substances and wants to eliminate them. If she cannot accomplish that herself the physician must create an artificial outlet in order to escape the harmful products."

Nature's way of getting rid of these harmful substances is through hemorrhages, inflammation, abscesses and other skin eruptions. The simplest means of cooperating with nature in her attempt to rid the body of these harmful substances is to go on a 100% raw food diet or a total fast, using only potable drinking water. Both are effective but the 100% raw food diet will probably be more effective because it will supply the required nutrients to the body while the body is healing itself and eliminating accumulations of toxic substances.

The medical men come along and use such things as aspirin, cortisone, prednisone and other modern drugs to relieve pain. They also use heat, massage or blistering plasters on the painful spot. Spanish fly is sometimes used as a blistering plaster. Also, irritating liniments such as croton oil, Sloan's liniment or Absorbine Jr. are used.

Here is a medical doctor, a rare one indeed, who in his

popular book on arthritis recommends a diet for arthritics . . . but just listen to this diet!

For breakfast, he suggests strong, black coffee with sugar; and a soft boiled egg with toast and butter. For lunch, he recommends two sandwiches on toast, fresh rolls or fresh sour rye bread, sandwiches made with ham or some other tender meat. Then, if you want something to drink, he suggests carbonated water, tea with lemon and sugar, sour milk, yogurt or good, black coffee. For dinner, he recommends strong beef or chicken soup with noodles, rice or similar farinaceous products. Then he says that the principle food should be meat, tender and well prepared.

He goes on to tell us — and just listen to this — that the fear of fried meat is not justified if one uses good cooking fat such as butter, lard, chicken fat or goose fat. Frying brings out the special flavor of meat better than broiling or boiling. It agrees particularly with the hyperacid sensitive stomach.

Then this highly respected medical genius goes on to tell us that fish as a substitute for meat is not recommended for the weak stomach, as it is more greasy and experience has shown that it is harder for many persons to digest than meat. He suggests that if fish is used it should be moderately spiced. He stresses that spicing is important because it helps to stimulate and support the digestive powers.

With a medically recommended diet like that, no wonder the medics say diet cannot help arthritis! This may also indicate why I say if you want to be healthy, you must stay as far away from medical doctors as humanly possible!

This selfsame doctor also tells us that since arthritis is a metabolic disturbance and the system is overcharged with irritants and waste products, correction of the faulty metabolism is of fundamental importance. The most effective way of cleaning the system has been and still is purging, with or without adequate dieting. Hence, the old medical axiom . . . He who purges well, cures well.

Galen, one of the really great medical men of all times, reports that he was able to cure the most advanced cases of arthritis, in addition to many other diseases, through purgation only. If he could cure the disease by that method, why can't the present day doctors do it? The answer is obvious . . . Galen never cured them in the first place. No doubt the continued purgation eventually removed the patient as well.

The following is a letter I received from a friend of mine who is a qualified medical doctor in good standing:

"Enclosed you will find a list of drugs I've just received from Medical Economics publication. But not all those drugs are used in various forms of arthritis.

"The list I sent you before was from a friend of mine, a Rheumatologist, a so-called specialist in the treatment of rheumatism in various forms. Believe me he does not cure them and that's for sure. Most of the drugs that you will read about in the list are just pain killers, nothing more. Most of the medications are combinations with codeine. Empirin compound contains codeine and all of these drugs, as I said before, have adverse side-effects. In fact, there is no drug that is free from side-effects and you know that.

"So the internist has nothing to offer. But, of course, he wouldn't tell his patients that. That is why I said in my previous letter to you that they neglect their patients to a degree that most of them end up on the operating table and, again, they are worse than before. The general public has tremendous faith, an unshakable faith in M.D.'s. They think they are some kind of gods.

"Here are the drugs they use:

"Corticosteroid, hydroxychloroquine, phenylbutozone,

indomethacin, gold compound, sodium salicylate and aspirin.

"All these drugs have terrific side-effects.

"In my estimation drug therapy was never any good or had any beneficial effects in any disease.

(Signed) N.I.B., M.D."

From the book, "Arthritis; Related Disorders," under the sub-heading, "Treatment," we quote:

"Therapy in rheumatoid arthritis with currently available medication is not curative. Proper management requires thorough understanding of the natural history of the disease. It also demands complete cooperation by the patient for many months or years, with realization of the aims, limitations and potential hazards of the medications involved. Because spontaneous remissions are frequent, management should be planned so as not to hamper the occurrence of a remission.

"**Rest and nutrition:** A patient with active rheumatoid arthritis needs rest periods during the day. but prolonged bed rest should be avoided because it aggravates the muscle wasting and negative nitrogen and Ca metabolism associated with the disease. Adequate nutrition should be maintained.

"**Counterirritants and salicylates:** Pain, which is caused by the inflammatory process, must be at least partially relieved before any measures to restore function can be instituted. Analgesia with narcotics is dangerous in this chronic disease and ineffectual in relieving pain. The anti-inflammatory property of salicylate (aspirin or sodium salicylate) is the backbone of antirheumatic management. It should be given in doses that achieve the desired effect (0.6 Gm. or more orally 4 times/day) or produce symptoms of early toxicity (e.g. tinnitus and nausea), and then adjusted to tolerance. When stiffness is the sole complaint during periods of low-grade activity, local heat and counterirritants can be effective.

"Only if a program of adequate nutrition, rest, local counterirritants and salicylates fails after a substantial trial (viz., 3 to 6 mo.) should more potentially hazardous medication be employed.

"**Gold compounds:** These are usually given in association with salicylates. Water-soluble gold compounds should be employed; colloidal gold has proved ineffectual. The usual dosage schedule consists of 25 to 50 mg./wk. I.M. until a total of 0.5 to 1.5 Gm. has been given. To determine tolerance to the drug, the initial dose should be 10 mg. When (or if) remission occurs, a relapse usually appears in the next 2 to 5 yr. if no further gold is administered. It is hoped that with prolonged administration of 25 to 50 mg. every 3 to 4 wk. remissions can be sustained. In general, in far-advanced stages with pronounced joint destruction and slight remaining inflammatory reaction, little is to be gained by the use of gold salts. Because of their toxic effects, gold compounds are contraindicated in those with present or past hepatic or renal disease, or with blood dyscrasia, and in acute systemic lupus erythematosus.

"Toxic reactions are ascribed to sensitivity to the compound or its vehicle, or to heavy metal toxicity. They include pruritis, dermatitis, stomatitis, vague gastrointestinal discomfort, albuminaria with a nephrotic syndrome, hematuria, agranulocytosis, thrombopenia with purpura, and aplastic anemia. When any of these manifestations appear, gold should be discontinued. *Before receiving gold,* the patient should have a complete urinalysis, a total and differential W.B.C., and an estimation of the number of platelets on the smear, with an actual count if they seem scarce. These tests should be repeated before each injection during the 1st mo., thereafter every 2 or 3 wk. during gold therapy. Eosinophilia greater than 4% may precede appearance of a rash. Pruritis almost always precedes the rash and is a danger signal. Dermatitis can range in severity from a single eczematous patch to generalized eruption with complete exfoliation, and death. Minor toxic manifestations (such as mild pruritis without a rash) may be eliminated by withholding treatment temporarily and resuming gold therapy cautiously. However, if toxic symptoms progress, not only should gold be withheld, but also the patient should be treated with dimercaprol or a corticosteroid. If hemopoietic toxicity develops, it is not safe to temporize. Gold should be withdrawn immediately and dimercaprol begun, preferably in hospital.

"**Phenylbutazone:** This drug, which has an anti-inflammatory effect, should be used only if the aforementioned therapy fails. It generally is given in a dosage of 100 mg. orally 4 times/day with reduction, if possible, to a maintenance level of 100 mg. 1 or 2 times/day. Although it satisfactorily controls the symptoms of rheumatoid spondylitis, its effectiveness in peripheral joint disease is not uniform. For this reason, and because of its severe toxic side effects (ulcerogenic, Na and water retention, dermatitis, stomatitis, agranulocytosis), it is not used to any major extent in rheumatoid arthritis.

"**Chloroquine:** This agent, with a mild anti-inflammatory effect, controls symptoms of active rheumatoid arthritis. However, its efficacy for this purpose has not been evaluated fully. Toxic side effects usually are mild, the most serious being corneal opacity, generally reversible. However, irreversible retinal degeneration has been attributed to chloroquine. The drug usually is given in an initial dosage of 250 mg./day orally with the evening meal; therapy for 1 to 3 mo. is required for effectiveness.

"**Indomethacin:** This unique antirheumatic drug shows

analgesic, anti-inflammatory and antipyretic activity; unlike corticosteroids, it has no effect on pituitary or adrenal function. It is effective in both rheumatoid arthritis and rheumatoid spondylitis. In these usually *chronic* disorders the initial dosage is 25 mg., 2 or 3 times/day, orally, with food or immediately after meals. If the response is inadequate, the daily dosage is increased by 25 mg. at about *weekly* intervals until a satisfactory response is obtained, or until a dosage of 150 to 200 mg./day is reached. Further increasing the dosage probably will not prove effective. If adverse reactions develop as the dosage is increased, it should be decreased to a tolerated level and so maintained for 3 to 4 wk. If an adequate response has not then been obtained, the daily dosage gradually is increased by 25 mg. at about weekly intervals to 150 to 200 mg./day.

"For patients with **acute** rheumatoid arthritis or **acute exacerbations** of chronic, one should increase the dosage **daily** by 25 mg. until a satisfactory response is obtained or a total daily dosage of 150 to 200 mg. is reached. If adverse effects develop as the dosage is increased, it should be reduced to a tolerated level for 2 or 3 days and then gradually increased by 25 mg. every few days as tolerated. After the acute phase of the disease is controlled, it is often possible to reduce the daily dosage of indomethacin gradually to a maintenance level of 75 to 100 mg./day.

"The most frequent adverse reactions associated with indomethacin are headache, dizziness, lightheadedness and gastrointestinal disturbances such as nausea, anorexia, vomiting, epigastric distress, abdominal pain, or diarrhea. The Central Nervous System effects are often transient and frequently disappear with continued treatment or after reduction of dosage; occasionally they are of such severity that therapy must be discontinued. Patients with significant

C.N.S. symptoms should not operate automotive equipment or engage in hazardous occupations. The gastrointestinal effects may be minimized by giving the drug immediately after meals or with food. If gastrointestinal bleeding occurs, the drug should be stopped. Indomethacin should not be given to patients with active peptic ulcer, gastritis, or ulcerative colitis, and should be used with caution if there is a past history of these disorders.

"**Adrenocortical steroids:** When the foregoing therapy is ineffective in controlling the inflammatory process and when the situation is rapidly and progressively worsening, adrenocortical steroids may be given. Because none of the medications available (including steroids) prevents articular cartilage destruction, this graded approach using the least toxic medications first, then progressing to more toxic agents, can be followed with least hazard to the patient. If steroid therapy is required, it must be remembered that rheumatoid arthritis can be active for many years. When the disease is active, intermittent use of steroids has not been effective because severe rebound phenomena appear following their withdrawal, requiring readministration of steroids for relief. Because of the side effects of these drugs, they should be given in adult rheumatoid arthritis only after careful and sometimes prolonged observation with less potentially hazardous medicaments. . . .

"**Intra-articular hormonal treatment:** Injections of hydrocortisone acetate or hydrocortisone *tertiary*-butylacetate have been of temporary help in controlling local synovitis. From 25 to 50 mg. may be injected into larger joints, and 5 to 20 mg. into small joints. The specific local effect usually lasts only 5 to 10 days. Alternatively, the 21-phosphate preparations of prednisolone or dexamethasone or the *tertiary*-butylacetate forms of these corticosteroids may be employed in appropriate dosage. Beneficial effects may be maintained if the joint is not traumatized during the period of temporary improvement and if other areas of rheumatoid arthritis are being adequately controlled, systemically or otherwise.

"**Technic of intra-articular injection:** Before attempting paracentesis of a joint, the physician should be familiar with its anatomic features, and may find an X-ray or a diagram helpful. The optimum approach is on the extensor surface where the synovial pouch is closest to the skin, and as remote as possible from major nerves, arteries, or veins. . . .

"The skin must be fully cleansed, thorough aseptic precautions being observed. If marked effusion is present, it may not be necessary to infiltrate the tissues with procaine, as introduction of the needle is relatively painless. In some persons, brief spraying of the area with ethyl chloride is sufficient.

"The aspirating needle seldom need be larger than 20 gauge. It should be inserted quickly through the skin, subcutaneous tissue, joint capsule and synovial membrane. If diagnosis has been established and paracentesis is only for treatment, the aspirating syringe then may be detached, allowing the needle to remain in place.

"The desired amount of the preferred corticosteroid preparation is drawn into a small syringe, which is then attached to the aspirating needle and the medicament injected into the cavity. The site of insertion is covered with a sterile dressing. Weight-bearing joints may require an elastic bandage to support the now relaxed joint capsule.

"**Exercise, physiotherapy and surgery:** Whatever regimen has been followed, prevention of flexion contractures and attempts at restoration of muscular strength and mass can be instituted once the symptoms of rheumatoid arthritis (pain, fatigue and weakness) are modified. All the physiotherapeutic measures available should be used. It is emphasized that splinting a joint facilitates atrophy of the associated muscle and does not prevent destruction of cartilage. Passive exercise should be given carefully within the limits of pain. In order to prevent the occurrence of contractures, it is best employed before the acute inflammatory process is controlled and before active exercises can be instituted. Active exercise, the only way to restore muscle mass, should be urged when feasible, but limited in extent so as not to produce excessive fatigue. Self-help devices have enabled many patients with severe debilitating rheumatoid arthritis to perform activities essential to daily living.

"If flexion contractures have become established, they require orthopedic measures such as gentle stretching by either wedged casts or manipulation. In some instances, surgical intervention is necessary for correction. However, these patients do not respond well to operative procedure while the disease is active."

Here I am giving a list of drugs that are generally used in the treatment of arthritis in its various forms:

Antiarthritics

Ascodeen-30 (Burroughs Wellcome), Ascriptin (Rorer), Aspercreme (Sperti), Azolid (USV Pharmaceutical), Azolid A (USV Pharmaceutical) Butazolidin (GEIGY), Butazolidin alka (GEIGY), Cama Inlay-Tabs (Dorsey), Celestone Soluspan Suspension (Schering), Celestone Syrup and Tablets (Schering), Cirin (Zemmer), Decadron Elixir (Merck Sharp & Dohme), Decadron Phosphate Injection (Merck, Sharpe & Dohme), Decadron Tablets (Merck, Sharpe & Dohme), Delta-Dome Tablets (Dome), Deronil Tablets (Schering), Ecotrin (Smith Kline & French), Empirin Compound (Burroughs Wellcome), Empirin Compound w/Codeine

Phosphate Nos. 1, 2, 3 & 4 (Burroughs Wellcome), Gaysal (Geriatric), Ger-O-Foam (Geriatric), Hyalex (Miller), Indocin (Merck Sharp & Dohme), Kenacort (Tablets & Syrup) (Squibb), Kenalog-10 Injection (Squibb), Kenalog-40 Injection (Squibb), Kengesin (Kenwood), Meticortelone Acetate Aqueous Suspension (Schering), Meticorten Tablets (Schering), Motrin Tablets (Upjohn), Os-Cal-Gesic (Marion), Ossonate Plus Capsulets (Marcen), Oxalid (USV Pharmaceutical), Pabalate (Robins), Pabalate-SF (Robins), Pabirin Buffered Tablets (Dorsey), Plaquenil Sulfate (Winthrop), Solganal (Schering), Sterazolidin (GEIGY), Tandearil (GEIGY).

Antigout

Anturane (GEIGY), Azolid (USV Pharmaceutical), Benemid (Merck Sharp & Dohme), Butazolidin (GEIGY), Butazolidin alka (GEIGY), ColBENEMID (Merck Sharp & Dohme), Colchicine Ampoules (Lilly), Colchicine Tablets (Lilly), Hyalex (Miller), Indocin (Merck Sharp & Dohme), Oxalid (USV Pharmaceutical), Tandearil (GEIGY), Zyloprim (Burroughs Wellcome).

From an article that appeared in the magazine, Science Digest, under the heading, "U.S. — USSR joint attack on arthritis", we quote:

"The U.S. and the USSR are combining forces to fight arthritis by establishing a rapid exchange of information, elimininating duplication of research, and organizing joint conferences and symposiums both in the United States and in the Soviet Union. The U.S. specialists are especially interested in the Soviet three-stage method of treatment of rheumatoid arthritis. The first stage consists of a 'shock' treatment of a patient with medical preparations. After this the patient is released from the hospital and is placed under the care of a local doctor who continues to prescribe smaller doses of medication. The third stage includes physiotherapy and water

163

fortification. They are also examining the Soviet surgical methods which are used when the changes in the joints are irreversible. The most important problem being tackled by both countries is the cause of rheumatic diseases and what prompts their development. . . ."

This article was of great interest to me because it clearly displays the fact that the medical profession is no different whether it is in Russia, the United States, Canada or Great Britain. They must play according to the rules . . . they must stay true to form. In other words, the medical profession must play at being God.

Instead of telling people plainly that their diet needs correcting — thus immediately preventing their arthritic condition from growing worse — they prefer to allow them to remain in ignorance. They treat these people in various ways that can never bring them any benefits . . . but which keep their pockets empty.

I am sure that the medical profession all over the world must realize the role that cooked food, refined food, white sugar and such play in arthritis, but they refuse to see . . . and "None are so blind as those who will not see."

A doctor must be a doctor. He cannot make the cure or the remedy simple and natural because that would not enhance his Godly image.

From my actual observations on the scene in Russia, the arthritis situation seems to be as bad or worse there than it is in America. The reason? While they do not have the high degree of chemical food additives and food processing in the USSR that they do in America, they also do not eat as many raw salads as we do. Yes, I found it difficult, if not impossible, to get a good salad dish in the USSR. Therefore, I believe their incidence of arthritis is as high or even higher than that in the United States.

Please read carefully this excerpt from the autobiography of the late E. F. Benson, entitled 'Final Edition,' which was published in 1940 because I contend that this bit of writing more or less proves what I say about the general treatment of arthritis throughout America:

"Most people of middle age are liable to rheumatic twinges, and though disquisitions on ailments are apt to be boring, I take that risk in hope that my long experience (I celebrate the completion of twenty glorious years of crippling processes very soon) may divert or encourage other wayfarers on that dreary road. . . . These twinges much annoyed me, for I had been a skilled and active denizen of skating rinks and golf links and tennis courts, impervious to fatigue, and I regarded such threatened limitations as an offense against the liberty of the subject.

"So I hastened to consult an eminent general practitioner, who after flexings and extensions, solemnly bound a strip of adhesive plaster round the troublesome hip joint which came off in my bath. I knew he used suggestion with his patients and concluded that this was an appeal to my mind. But my mind must have been in an unreceptive mood: the treatment had no effect.

"It would be as tedious to follow the progress of this repulsive ailment as it was to suffer it. Like a clock of which the long pointer remains stationary till a minute is completed, it paused and then registered a perceptible advance. Activity diminished and pain, which I abominate, increased.

"Firmly resolved to get rid of it, I scoured the medical cantonments of London. I went alike to notable regular physicians and quacks. I returned to my friend of the sticking-plaster, who now advised tonics and a liberal consumption of oranges. He said there was no need to take an X-ray because he knew what it would show.

"Another gave me a course of atophan; another colonized my colon with hordes of the Bacillus bulgaricus. When that region (such was the strategy) was securely held by this Army Corps, they would march and maneuver and inflict crushing defeats on the injurious bacilli of disease. I took great interest in this war. For two years I was a very diligent Colonial Minister, and kept adding brigades of Bacillus bulgaricus to my garrisons, but they never seemed to win a single engagement.

"Another doctor injected something radioactive into my thigh; another some potion of dead bacilli into my arm. Another drove iodine into the hip by means of an electric current; another prescribed a course of iodine taken internally in increasing doses up to the maximum and then in diminished doses, till I arrived at the precise point in every sense, at what I had started. Another prescribed massage, another a system of physical exercises.

"I wallowed in brown mud, I drank the waters of Bath, and had some healthy teeth extracted. I had a course of intensive X-ray, alone in a room full of shining black pipes and buzzing mechanisms; it was figuring in some nightmare picture by Syme. Never in my life have I pursued a quest with such unfaltering devotion. The zeal of the Lords of Harley Street ate me up.

"The quacks, if I may call them so without libel, were equally enterprising and empirical. I took herbal teas and sat in tepid baths. For a long time I wore a band of small crystals, which I take to have been glass, around my neck, and 'radioactive pads,' which I take to have been flannel, over my hips, for both were now giving trouble. I carried a little tubular cardboard case, hermetically sealed and very heavy for its size, in my trouser pocket. One day I dropped it on the floor, the case was fractured and inside was a small bottle of

166

quicksilver.

"I had a course — perhaps I ought to class this among scientific treatments — of Christian Science. The healer, a most charming fellow, gave me something by Mrs. Eddy to read, while he tuned in, as it were, by dipping into her textbook, *Christian Science and the Key to the Scriptures.* He then closed his book and gave me mental treatment; that is to say, he absorbed himself in the conviction that disease had not any real existence, with special application to me, I warned him that I was not yet a convert, but he said that did not matter; faithless folk, who had a false claim that they were ill, could be cured just as well as believers. This astonished me, for I had understood that in the miracles of healing recorded in the Gospels the faith of the patient was a condition of his cure.

"These treatments overlapped. I might be wearing my 'radioactive pads' at Droitwich or my necklace at Bath. They all ran the same course, cradled in high optimism and gently expiring in complete failure. But I wanted to get well, and was prepared to do anything, however preposterous, in search of this consummation. Indeed, I think it would have been very foolish not to have been so foolish, for who could tell?

"From time to time these practitioners cheered me up by telling me that I was walking more easily, which was not the case, for when at last one of them suggested that an X-ray skiagraph should be taken, it showed osteoarthritis in an advanced stage, and irreparable damage already done."

Here is the best advice the medical profession can offer an arthritic sufferer, according to a medical column in the Chicago Tribune, Saturday, May 31, 1975, entitled "How to Keep Well" by T. R. Van Dellen, M.D.:

"A Man from River Forest writes: 'I am 72 years old and have osteoarthritis all thru my system. Would moist treatment — such as the use of hot or wet towels or bathing in a whirlpool — or deep dry heat give me the most relief?'

"You'll have to try both and see which gives you more relief. As a rule, moist heat is better than dry heat.

"A warm bath, with or without a whirlpool attachment, should lessen your distress. Also, a hot towel kept warm by a heating pad or infrared lamp works very well when only one or two joints are involved.

. "Aspirin in large enough doses — be sure you are being supervised by a physician — is an excellent pain reliever for your condition. As a step to cut down on the inflammation, injection of a steroid medication directly into the joints by your physician may give added relief. If these measures do not help, your physician may choose to administer, on a trial basis, an oral antiinflammatory drug such as phenylbutazone, or a new agent, Motrin (ibuprofen).

"If then your pain remains pinpointed and unabating and you are otherwise in good health, then you might think of seeing an orthopedic surgeon. Considering the orthopedist's armamentarium, almost any joint in the body can be replaced with an artificial one made out of steel or teflon. The era of an artificial man nearly has arrived."

From my extensive study of the medical view and treatment of arthritis, it is obvious that they see arthritis as something you have to learn to live with. They can do nothing for you except give you drugs and various other treatments . . . but none are in any way curative. Of course, this means using various drugs, surgery, X-rays or radium that will perhaps lessen your pain or render you oblivious to pain and in this way you will live with your arthritis and spend the rest of your life trying to minimize the aches, the pains and the suffering.

Now when I say this, I say it without fear of

contradiction by any medical man in America. I say it because it is true, I say it because it is obvious and has been proven. To my way of thinking this is a peculiar if not ridiculous or even a deplorable attitude. What the medical profession is doing is fencing with the poor arthritic sufferer to minimize his pain for a lifetime and as arthritis now strikes in youth, it could mean spending 50, 60 or more years in various degrees of pain.

As I have mentioned elsewhere in the book, if you suffer from arthritis don't worry too much about dying from it because it is certain that no one dies from arthritis. I am not even sure that it shortens your life. However, you do suffer the twinges and pains of the disease.

Some unusual methods of treating arthritis are these received in letters from some of my readers:

"You may not agree with me but I must tell you my arthritic story — at 18 I started with swelled knees. In a short time it disappeared, then as I grew older I really developed arthritis. Yes, the doctor prescribed aspirin, but I do not like to take pills and medicine or shots of any kind. So I surprisingly found sea water at the Natural Health store, 3 tablespoons in a quart of water, and believe it or not I am practically cured. For three months I could not find it in the store so I know it works because backwards I went. Then I started taking it again and so help me it did help. Now at 68 I am in excellent health. You asked me for an experience so here it is for what it might mean to you. I also live pretty close to many of your recommendations.

"Respectfully,

G . I . B ."

"I see in the Provoker you are asking for testimonies on arthritis. I had sciatic rheumatism for years and by using a raw potato in my shirt pocket for a month I got rid of it and never had it since and that was 30 years ago.

"I had arthritis of the left knee and after trying various remedies I cured it by drinking raw potato juice.

"Yours truly,

O.S."

"I am reading the Provoker from my brother. It is a very fine eye opener. In May-June copy you ask your readers to send you any information they have on arthritis for the book you are writing.

"The Sure Cure for arthritis is the following recipe:

1 Cup or more water

50-100 violet leaves (Can use stems and blossoms if in blossom)

25 or more mint leaves (tips and blossoms if in blossom)

2-3 stalks of celery cut in little pieces

1 or 2 stalks of rhubarb cut in small pieces. If rhubarb is not available, juice of 2-3 lemons

Sweeten with tablespoon of honey.

Put in blender until liquid. More water or any fruit juice may be added. Put in jar and store under refrigeration.

Take 1/2 cup morning and 1/2 cup in the evening. Guaranteed arthritis gone in one week to 10 days.

"Sincerely yours,

A. G."

"I read in a catholic magazine about a lady being cured of arthritis by taking Certo that you use for making jelly — 49c a bottle — 3 spoonsful a day. Well, I decided to try it, too — yes, I took 1 bottle and 6 spoonsful from the second bottle and that was all — no more pain in my fingers and hands. I am entirely cured — I have not taken any now for at least 2 months and more women say they, too, have been cured.

"Try it and find out for yourself.

"Sincerely yours,

C.D."

Here are some remedies I came across when doing my book, "Proven Herbal Remedies":

ARTHRITIS AND MALNUTRITION

PLANT: Lucerne or Alfalfa   *Medigo sativa*
WHERE FOUND: Europe and America; wherever cattle are raised.
PART USED: Whole Herb
ACTION: Alterative, nutritive
DISSERTATION: Known generally as alfalfa. It is best known as one of the finest of all grasses for cattle. Its nutritive value has been recognized for centuries. Widely used for arthritis, where the powdered herb is taken with cider vinegar and honey: one teaspoonful of each in a glass of water. Has long been used as a strengthening and weight adding tonic.

Dioscorides back in the first century prescribed a concoction that he called 'OXYMEL' for the treatment of arthritis, epilepsy and snake-bite. 'OXYMEL' literally translated means sour honey, and the first English translator wrote it as Vinegar-Honey.

ARTICULAR STIFFNESS

PLANT: Poison Oak   *Rhis toxicodendron*
WHERE FOUND: North America
PART USED: Leaves
ACTION: Irritant, narcotic, stimulant
DISSERTATION: Valuable in articular stiffness and acute

171

rheumatism. Also has been used with success in the treatment of obstinate skin diseases and in small doses is an excellent sedative for the nervous system.

METHOD: Liquid extract

DOSAGE: 5 to 30 drops

Thousands swear that wearing a copper bracelet or wearing copper in their shoes to contact the skin has brought marvelous curative effects to arthritis. As a matter of fact, as of this writing there is a medical researcher at the University of Akron who is doing work on the subject and he seems to think there is something about copper that affects arthritis. I am trying to get some more information on the subject but at the present time there is not much available.

CHAPTER 25

NEW DRUGS

Here I would like to quote a recent magazine article entitled, "Killing Arthritis Pain":

"Stronger and safer drugs to ease arthritis pain are now getting their first tests in humans.

"The new drugs, called 'chelates,' are actually well-known pain killers and anti-inflammatory agents with traces of copper added.

"Dr. John R. J. Sorenson of the University of Cincinnati College of Medicine reported to the American Chemical Society: 'The data, to date, demonstrate that . . . the copper chelates, or complexes prepared from them, have more anti-inflammatory activity than the clinically used antiarthritic drugs.'

"The new drugs are also agents against ulcers — a big advantage since present pain killers, including aspirin, carry the risk of ulcers and intestinal bleeding.

"It may be a year or more before the new drugs are approved by the Food and Drug Administration."

Perhaps those fanatics who recommend the use of the copper bracelets are not as crazy as some people think they are. I reserve my opinion. Some people wear copper bracelets

173

on both wrists and some even wear them on their ankles and they claim their arthritis is relieved. Who knows? Maybe there is a good logical reason why those bracelets work. My attitude is that since people do wear jewelry, gadgets, trinkets and baubles on their arms, legs, neck and body . . . why not wear copper bracelets or rings if there is a chance they may have healing qualities?

Here is some data from a report in a California newspaper, dated April 2, 1975:

"On the horizon are 80 new drugs to relieve the pain, stiffness and inflammation of joints in rheumatoid arthritis. . . .

"Progress against arthritis 'has been terribly slow, despite all sorts of approaches,' says Dr. Paul Plotz, senior investigator of the Arthritis and Rheumatism Branch of the National Institute of Arthritis, Metabolism and Digestive Disease — NIAMDD.

"So arthritis is counted among the 'stalled diseases' requiring more effort and insights to bring it under control.

"Fifty million Americans, one in four, have some form of arthritis, and 20 million, one in 10, have it so severely they need medical care, says the Arthritis Foundation in New York City. Specialists now count 100 different arthritic conditions causing aches and pains in joints and connective tissue.

"Some 3.5 million Americans are disabled by arthritis, and the economic cost, including $3.5 billion lost in wages of people who could otherwise be productive, is put at $9 billion a year.

"Most serious, most painful and most crippling is rheumatoid arthritis, causing inflammation of joints, with women hit three times more often than men. About five million Americans are victims.

"Bacteria or viruses have long been suspect as possible

causes of rheumatoid arthritis. Cultures taken from joints have shown unusual organisms, but none has yet been proven to be either an important or specific cause of this woeful disease.

"The search for infectious agents goes on. For if one (or more) is found, vaccines might be developed to prevent rheumatoid arthritis and the numerous other arthritic conditions.

"Other researchers are studying whether the fire of rheumatoid arthritis is lighted by something going haywire in the body's normally protective immune system, with some unusual reaction turning antibodies against joints or other tissues.

"Just what happens in this complexity is beginning to be pieced together, says Dr. Charles W. Sisk, former medical director of the Arthritis Foundation. 'Researchers are very close to being able to translate basic new knowledge into treatment.'

"Citing an example, Sisk says that certain white blood cells, the lymphocytes that normally fight infection, are suspected as one trigger of arthritis inflammation.

"In one experiment by Drs. Harold Paulus and James Peter of the University of California at Los Angeles, billions of these white cells were withdrawn each day from rheumatoid arthritis patients, through tubes placed in their necks.

"With the white cells diminished, most patients felt less pain, less swelling and tenderness of joints, perhaps because the lymphocyte system was temporarily exhausted. Benefits lasted for months.

"Research is pointing toward definite genetic factors in at least some forms of arthritis, Sisk says, and these may shed some insight into how the immune system goes wrong. Certain genes may produce antigens or substances that stimulate antibodies that enter into the inflammation process.

"In treatment, aspirin has long been the white knight of drugs combating arthritic pain, and remains so.

"Cortisone made a dramatic appearance more than 20 years ago, enabling some severely disabled people to walk again. But now, two decades later, many patients treated with cortisone or allied hormone or steroid drugs, appear no better off, and in some cases they are worse off, Plotz says.

"Six years ago, a totally different drug, indomethacin, appeared. It is not in the hormone family, but is in a class of chemicals that counteracts inflammation. It has to be monitored carefully for possible adverse effects on blood components.

"Now, a number of drugs have been fashioned, starting with the indomethacin family, that promise fewer side effects.

"Today, if drugs fail surgery often helps by providing artificial joints for crippled originals.

"Surgical replacement of various joints has increased tenfold in the last 10 years, says Sisk. Perhaps 40,000 Americans each year are enabled now to walk again with artificial hip joints.

"Fingers grotesquely twisted by arthritis are being restored in surgery pioneered by Dr. A. B. Swanson of Grand Rapids, Mich., and others. Silicone rubber is implanted to replace tissue, with the implants soon becoming surrounded by healthy tissue. Patients go back to using their hands for sewing, typing, the piano, all manner of tasks, and play. Toe joints also are replaced.

"Silicone rubber additionally is being molded into new elbow and wrist joints, and new shoulder and knee replacements. This research is in various stages of development.

" 'The knee is more complicated than the hip,' Sisk says,

'but the biomechanisms of motions and muscle functions are being worked out. Joe Namath (the New York Jets quarterback with injured knees) could have new knees now if only the state of the art for replacement of knees were like it is now for hips.'

"For all the misery arthritis causes, the federal budget for research into it is only $14 million a year now, up from $11.5 million in 1970. The Arthritis Foundation raises $10 million annually for research fellowships, referral centers, and educational efforts.

"Recent cutbacks in research money have hurt with 'good people having to close their laboratories,' Plotz says. 'Answers will come from basic research, not from research administratively directed to find answers. If, for example, we understood the immune response itself, it would be a big step toward control not only of arthritis but other diseases as well.'

"Sisk calls for more training of specialists in rheumatology."

This only helps to prove what I have said before, that the medical profession knows nothing about the cause of arthritis or the disease itself, yet there is a rise in actual cash flow into the medical men's coffers . . . more than two billion dollars annually. I say that is pretty good for a disease that they cannot cure, don't know the cause of and cannot even help . . . except to worsen the condition.

I claim that, as usual, the medical profession is looking away from the true cause of the disease because to find the answer would mean the loss of more than two billion dollars annually. The medical profession can't afford that loss and, therefore, they are hunting for a bacteria or virus or some such thing, which they know they'll never find, as being the cause of arthritis.

From a newspaper article that appeared in the Miami Herald, May 18, 1975, we read of another new drug called Motrin:

"The new prescription drug, Motrin, is being turned out at a million tablets a day from the Upjohn company's Kalamazoo, Mich., plant and that is still not enough to meet demand after only seven months on the market. An Upjohn spokesman said that it will be late summer or fall before the drug, which was introduced last October, is produced in quantity to fill all prescriptions."

This drug is supposed to be more effective than aspirin, and produces fewer adverse effects.

Now I want to quote from an advertisement that appeared in the Medical Post of April 1, 1975, for Alka Butazolidin mantle tablets manufactured by the Geigy Company. Read it and weep.

"Maximum Butazolidin benefits with minimum gastric upset in severe acute non-infectious conditions such as: severe osteoarthritis, acute superficial thrombophlebitis, acute attacks of gout, rheumatoid arthritis, ankylosing (rheumatoid) spondylitis, bursitis, peritendinitis, capsulitis. . . .

Dosage

"The recommended initial daily dose for arthritis, rheumatism and superficial thrombophlebitis is 3-6 tablets — patients experiencing an acute attack of gout may require up to 9 tablets per day. Alka Butazolidin should be taken in divided doses with meals. When improvement is obtained (generally in two or three days), the dose should be reduced to the lowest effective level. The maintenance level should not exceed 4 tablets per day. In the absence of a favourable response after a one week trial period, Alka Butazolidin administration should be discontinued. Alka Butazolidin mantle tablets have been specifically designed for patients with a sensitive gastrointestinal tract. . . .

Contraindications

"Alka Butazolidin is contraindicated in patients with a history of blood dyscrasia or drug allergy and in those with a history of symptoms of peptic ulcer. In addition, it should not be given to senile patients, to patients with clinical edema or to those with severe renal hepatic or cardiac disease. . . .

Precautions

"A careful history, physical examination and a complete blood count should be done before initiating therapy. Patients receiving this drug should be followed closely and should be warned to discontinue Alka Butazolidin and contact their physician immediately should any of the following signs and symptoms appear: fever, sore throat, lesions in the mouth, black or tarry stools, skin reactions or a sudden gain in weight. Patients undergoing long-term therapy should have blood counts done at regular intervals. Care should be taken when prescribing for the elderly. As with any drug, Alka Butazolidin should not be used during the first trimester of pregnancy unless in the opinion of the prescribing physician, the potential benefits outweigh the possible risks. . . .

Side Effects

"Nausea, vomiting, abdominal discomfort, formation or activation of peptic ulcer and sodium retention with edema are known to occur. Although rarely observed, hypersensitivity reactions, dermatological reactions and blood dyscrasias have been reported."

The above quote runs true for most of the drugs that are sold in North America today, yet the poor unsuspecting public knows little or nothing about it. While the doctor is informed about this the patient is seldom if ever informed about the side effects of the drug. This is because they are afraid that if you knew the risks involved, you would not take the prescribed drugs.

I have repeatedly claimed that the supposed cures for arthritis are invariably worse than the disease itself. It is becoming a genuine comedy of errors ... except, it is no comedy to those afflicted.

I wish I could reach the ears of the arthritis sufferers and tell them that the answer is a drastic change of diet along with a proper way of life and that they could relieve their pain and suffering and even regain their mobility.

The newspapers give free space to all of the new medical wonders ... but there is not a word to tell the sufferer that the true answers are through nutrition and a proper way of life.

How can I reach the sufferers and tell them that they don't have to be guinea pigs? They don't have to take these untested drugs and suffer the pain and agony these drugs cause, nor the pain and agony of the disease itself, if only they will lift up their eyes and see the truth.

CHAPTER 26

RAW FOOD

I was amazed — no, more than that, I was virtually astounded — no, better than that, I was thunderstruck when I learned about all the outlandish, bizarre and horrendous means and methods that have been used in trying to find a cure for arthritis . . . when the the most natural, the simplest and the safest method is being ignored.

Instead of taking a sane logical approach to reach their goal of freedom from pain and a return to good health, the arthritic sufferers take every possible turn, twist and curve that it is humanly possible to take. No, they just will not take the straight and narrow way that will lead them to good health and long life.

Furthermore, practically every other method of treating arthritis costs money, while the safe, sure, proper and most direct method doesn't cost anything. Maybe that is the answer. Perhaps they think it can't be any good if it doesn't cost money.

Well, I am going to tell you the proper way to conquer arthritis. As for a permanent cure, that will depend entirely upon you. If you continue to follow the proper way of life that I advocate, then the conquest will be permanent. If you deviate, then it will be a different story entirely. The choice is yours.

The answer to this great enigma is simply the proper way of life and a diet consisting of fresh vegetables, grains, fruits and nuts in the widest possible variety. The only proviso is that they must be eaten raw . . . unheated, untreated and uncooked. They must be eaten as close to the way nature made them as possible.

The most important foods for good health are the vegetables and I am quite certain that you could enjoy the best of health on a diet consisting of a wide variety of wholesome vegetables only. However, I usually recommend seeds and grains of all kinds because they are energy promotors and they are satisfying and tasty. Whereas a meal consisting of only vegetables may not be filling and may not stay with you very long, meaning you will have to eat more often, a meal including grains and seeds of various kinds will do both. They are filling and they will provide enough nutritive potency to last you for at least four hours and usually longer.

In my opinion fruits, which are the best tasting and the most pleasing of all nature's gifts, are not nearly as nourishing as vegetables and grains and while nuts are excellent food, there is always the tendency to overeat nuts. Overeating is just as bad as eating the wrong food so I am reluctant to advise the regular use of nuts in one's diet. If you do use nuts, never eat more than two ounces of shelled nuts at a time under any circumstances.

I have proven that you can live on a raw food diet more cheaply than the conventional meat and potato diet. Here I will give you as complete a list as possible of the various kinds of vegetables, grains and seeds, fruits and nuts. Most of them are available every day in the market places of America and they are comparatively inexpensive.

Some of the most popular vegetables are asparagus, green beans, broccoli, cabbage, celery, cress, endive, escarole, lettuce, parsley, peas, especially the edible podded peas, spinach, kale, mushrooms, beets, carrots, parsnips, radishes, turnips, kohlrabi, garlic, onions, leeks, chives, cucumber, egg plant, peppers, tomatoes, squash, okra, salsify, chicory, peanuts and chard.

Some seeds in widespread use are sunflower, pumpkin, wheat, barley, rye, oats, flax, sesame, millet, buckwheat, corn, lentils, garbanzo beans and rice.

Under fruits we have apple, pear, plum, peach, cherry, grape, apricot, orange, lemon, grapefruit, mulberry, watermelon, honeydew melon, canteloupe, spanish melon, crenshaw melon, red, black, gold and purple raspberries, strawberries, boysenberries, loganberries, gooseberries, black currants, red currants, mango, papaya, kumquat, persimmon and also many other semi-tropical and tropical fruit.

Some of the nuts are hazel or filbert, walnut, pecan, almond, Brazil, macadamia, pistachio, cashew, pignolia and hickory.

For all you doubting Thomases who are skeptical about the merits of a raw food diet and just can't believe that a raw food diet will work when all the physicians and healers in the world use drugs, medicines, herbs, potions, massage, manipulation and surgery, well, all you have to do is try it. I sincerely urge you to try a strictly 100% raw food diet, as I advocate, for 30 days. From that moment on you will never doubt the merit of raw food again. I say that a raw food diet is the most powerful healing force that exists on the face of the earth. All diseases crumble at its onslaught.

Here is a list of foods that many people think of as 'raw' but which have actually been heated, cooked or treated in some other way, which makes them non-nutritious: peanut butter, practically all dairy products, including butter, yogurt, ice cream, cream, cottage cheese, as well as other varieties of cheese, rolled oats, raw sugar, molasses, pasteurized honey, margarine, oils, soya flour, powdered milk, cashews and many other shelled nuts.

I took the trouble to mention these foods because so many people believe they are raw foods and I don't want them to suffer from any delusions and do themselves harm when they think they are benefitting themselves by eating them. Remember, all items on this list have been treated or heated in one form or another.

From Linda Clark's book entitled, "Get Well Naturally," we read:

"Dr. O. Stiner, an investigator for the Swiss Board of Health, in Berne, Switzerland, took a large number of guinea pigs off their normally raw diet and fed them food cooked in a pressure cooker. The animals developed softened teeth, gum disturbances, goiter, and anemia. When two teaspoons of pasteurized milk were added daily, arthritis appeared."

In my association with people I am frequently faced with a question like this, "If a raw food diet is so effective, then why doesn't the medical profession recommend this method of healing arthritis?"

My reply is always very clear and to the point, "Why not ask your medical doctors? No doubt they have very good personal reasons!"

At this point I would like to relate the old joke about the young, newly graduated son of a medic who took over his father's practice while he went on an extended vacation.

With great pride of achievement, the son told his father when he returned, "You know Mrs. Idlerich, the lady you have been treating for arthritis for over ten years ... well, she is now cured. I took her off the medication and put her on a mainly raw food diet for 30 days and she is almost as good as new."

Father replied, "It was the fees from Mrs. Idlerich that put you through college and I hoped she would put your sister through, too, but now you've loused things up."

I have asked a great many medical doctors why they don't recommend a raw food diet and the answer usually goes something like this, "It's nonsensical and ridiculous! How could a simple thing like one's food make any difference? Besides, all the great physicians in the world have been working on a means and method of cure for centuries without results."

Dorothy C. Hare, C.B.E., M.D., writing in the British journal, *Proceedings of the Royal Society of Medicine,* Vol. 30, 1936, describes the experiment at the Royal Free Hospital, in which 12 rheumatic patients were put on this 'raw food diet,' as she called it:

Breakfast: Porridge made of grated apple, soaked raw oatmeal, grated nuts, cream, fresh orange, tea with milk and cream.

Mid-morning: Tomato puree with lemon.

Dinner: Salad of lettuce, cabbage, tomato, root vegetables, salad dressing with oil, mixed fruit salad and cream.

Tea: Dried fruits, nuts and tea with milk and cream.

Supper: Fruit porridge, prune, apricot or apple, and salad dish with dressing.

Bedtime: Lemon and orange juice with hot water.

After two weeks, the following cooked foods were added to this diet: vegetable soup, one egg, two ounces of meat, two ounces of bacon, two ounces of bread and some butter, cheese and milk.

At no time during the weeks of the diet was any salt used on either the raw or the cooked foods. The raw oatmeal and the dried fruits were thoroughly soaked in water, the vegetables were shredded and the nuts were crushed or whole. All the food was prepared fresh for every meal and it was attractively served.

The results? Eight of the twelve patients began to feel better in from one to four weeks on this so-called raw food diet. Two of the patients improved noticeably for up to five or six weeks and then relapsed. The other two showed no improvement at all. In a follow-up, after the patients who improved had gone home, it was discovered that seven of them continued to improve to a marked degree.

One patient, who was 46 years old, had suffered for four years with occasional pain and swelling of the knees but for the three months before she was admitted to the hospital she had general pain and stiffness in the shoulders, arms, knees and legs. She had been in bed for ten weeks. There was fluid in both knee joints, with swelling and pain in other joints. She was discharged from the hospital after being on the diet for three weeks. She continued the diet and, after being on it for seven more weeks, she was free from all pain and was able to do her housework.

In commenting on the success of her diet, Dr. Hare remarked on the fact that the rawness of the food seemed to be the one outstanding factor that had brought about these results. The fact that the food was raw made a great impression on the patients themselves and on observers. She tells us that a Zurich physician, who used raw diets similar to this in treating rheumatism, claimed that the diet was successful "because of the absorption of the unaltered solar energy of plant life." Says Dr. Hare, "Science has so far revealed nothing . . . of this occult solar energy, as something apart from vitamin and chemical constituents (of food)."

Now for my remarks on the results of this experiment ....

Just imagine the tremendous results that would have been achieved had the diet been a genuinely raw food diet, the kind that I advocate. Soaked raw oatmeal usually means rolled oats and they are heat-treated in the rolling process. There is nothing raw about a cup of conventional tea with milk and cream that are pasteurized — and all dairy products used in hospitals are pasteurized. As for the tomato puree, I have never known canned tomato puree to be made without boiling and besides it contains a harmful chemical preservative. Salad dressings are invariably heated and the oil itself is processed by a heat treatment — even cold pressed oils are made under heat. Furthermore, virtually all commercial salad dressings contain monosodium glutamate, a known harmful substance banned from food by the Food and Drug Administration. You will also notice that they used lemon and orange juice with hot water. Then after two weeks, cooked foods were added: vegetable soup, eggs, meat, bacon, bread, butter, cheese and milk.

I suggest that, if they had put these patients on a 100% raw food diet for thirty days, the results would have been staggering! But, of course, they never would try a completely raw food diet because it would be successful and that would bring the medical profession's beliefs and convictions on drugs collapsing down around their heads. Yes, I firmly believe that the only reason the medical profession, the chiropractic profession, the osteopathic profession or any other healing profession does not advocate the raw food diet is simply because it would put them all out of business.

On occasion I come across some seriously interested people with high principles and a great love of humanity, who resent my nasty innuendos and serious castigations and lash out at me because they have been offended, saying "Mr. Tobe, do you suggest that all those thousands of dedicated healers, most of whom are members of the great and noble medical profession, are of such calibre that they would withhold a cure from people and watch them suffer . . . for money?"

I reply straightforwardly, "Yes, I mean precisely that! What else could be the reason they are standing by and watching millions of people suffer from arthritis while relief is so close at hand? Remember, arthritis is worth over two billion dollars a year to the medical profession alone, besides what it brings to other healers."

Can't you see that if a raw food diet ever became the 'in thing' it would spell economic disaster not only for the healing professions but for America. If all the people in America followed a raw food diet, the healing profession would have to close up shop. The doctors would all have to go out and get jobs as clerks, shippers, messengers, ditch diggers and such, which would not be nearly as remunerative as practising medicine. Does this logic sink into your cranium or do you need a surgeon to crack it open and implant a bit of good common horse sense?

Some of the rewarding things about a raw food diet for the treatment and cure of arthritis are: you don't need to go on a fast, you don't have to take enemas or laxatives, you don't have to take drugs or tranquilizers, you don't have to go in for the various manipulations including hot or cold baths or showers, you don't have to have your neck jerked or have massages, although I don't think there is anything wrong with being massaged. If you can afford to have a chiropractor or masseur treat you at regular intervals, I guess it is a pleasant interlude.

In order for you to better understand the effects of a raw food diet, I want you to read for yourself this report of an experiment by Dr. Paul Kouchakoff:

THE INFLUENCE OF FOOD COOKING ON THE BLOOD FORMULA OF MAN
by Paul Kouchakoff (Suisse), M.D.

of the

Institute of Clinical Chemistry, Lausanne, Switzerland

PROCEEDINGS: FIRST INTERNATIONAL CONGRESS OF MICROBIOLOGY, PARIS, 1930

Translated by Lee Foundation for Nutritional Reseach, Milwaukee 1, Wisconsin

The living organism is very sensitive to all harmful influences and reacts against them immediately.

We see this when we make an analysis of our blood during simple and infectious illnesses, when extraneous substances are introduced into our system, etc.

In such cases the number of white corpuscles changes and the correlation of percentage between them is disturbed. This is one of the indications of a pathological process going on in our system.

After every dose of food, we also observe a general augmentation of white corpuscles, and a change in the correlation of their percentage. This phenomenon has been considered, until now, a physiological one, and is called a digestive leukocytosis.

We use, for our food, raw foodstuffs, foodstuffs which have been altered by means of high temperature, and manufactured foodstuffs. How then does each one of these

foodstuffs separately act on our blood formula?

We find that, after taking raw foodstuffs, neither the number of white corpuscles nor the correlation of their percentage has changed. Ordinary unboiled drinking water, mineral water, salt, different green foodstuffs, cereals, nuts, honey, raw eggs, raw fish, fresh milk, sour milk, butter — in other words, foodstuffs in the state in which they exist in nature — belong to the group of those which do not call forth any infringement in our blood formula.

After the consumption of the same natural foodstuffs, altered by means of high temperature, we find that the general number of white corpuscles has changed, but the correlation of their percentage has remained the same.

After consumption of manufactured foodstuffs not only has the number of white corpuscles changed but also the correlation of percentage between them.

To this group belong sugar, wine, chocolate in tablet form, etc.

All our experiments have shown that it is not the quantity, but the quality of food which plays an important role in the alteration of our blood formula, and that 200 milligrams or even 50 milligrams of foodstuffs produce the same reaction as large doses of them. The experiments also show that the reaction in our blood takes place at the moment the food enters the stomach, while the preliminary mastication of food in the mouth softens the reaction.

We have already said that raw foodstuffs, altered by means of high temperature only, call forth an augmentation of the general number of white corpuscles.

Does this occur only when such foodstuffs are heated to boiling point, or is the same phenomenon called forth by lower temperatures?

It appears that every raw foodstuff has its own

temperature which must not be surpassed in heating, otherwise it loses its original virtues and calls forth a reaction in the system.

Ordinary drinking water, heated for half an hour to a temperature of 87 degrees (C.) does not change our blood, but this same water heated to 88 degrees (C.) changes it.

We have given the name 'critical temperature' to the highest degree of temperature at which a particular foodstuff can be cooked for half an hour in bain marie, and eaten, without changing our blood formula.

This critical temperature is not the same for all raw foodstuffs. It varies within a range of ten degrees. The lowest critical temperature for water is 87 degrees; for milk it is 88 degrees; for cereals, tomatoes, cabbage, bananas, 89 degrees; for pears, meat, 90 degrees; for butter, 91 degrees; for apples and oranges, 92 degrees; for potatoes, 93 degrees; for carrots, strawberries and figs, 97 degrees.

Our experiments show that it is possible to paralyze the action of a foodstuff, once its critical temperature is surpassed. There exist strictly definite laws for this, and the critical temperature plays the first role here.

If a cooked foodstuff is eaten along with the same product in a raw state there is no reaction.

The raw product has neutralized the action which this same product, with its critical temperature surpassed, would have called forth. In other words, the raw product has, so to say, re-established the virtues of the product altered by high temperature. Such a re-establishment is also possible when two different products have been absorbed, but with one condition; their critical temperature must either be the same, or else the critical temperature of the raw product must be higher than the critical temperature of the overheated one.

If the critical temperature of a raw product is lower than

that of the overheated one, the reaction is sure to take place; in this case, even the augmentation of the quantity of the raw products does not help.

This law remains the same when the raw product is mixed with several overheated ones of the same critical temperature.

If several cooked foodstuffs are taken, each with a different critical temperature, along with raw food, reaction takes place, even if the raw product has a higher critical temperature than that of any of the cooked foodstuffs.

Now we pass on to the 3rd group of foodstuffs, such as sugar, wine, etc. obtained by complicated manufacturing processes, and producing double reaction in our organism. These products may also be consumed without calling forth any reaction, but only when they are introduced into our organism conjointly with no less than two raw foodstuffs of a different critical temperature. Even one raw product has a beneficial influence on this 3rd group, and deprives them of one of their properties, namely the power of altering the correlation of percentage of the white corpuscles.

As regards the proportions in which raw products must be added to cooked foods, there is an irreducible minimum. For water, for example, it is 50%.

CONCLUSIONS

After over 300 experiments on ten individuals of different age and sex, we have come to the following conclusions:

1. The augmentation of the number of white corpuscles and the alteration of the correlation of the percentage between them which takes place after every consumption of food, and which was

192

considered until now as a physiological phenomenon, is, in reality, a pathological one. It is called forth by the introduction into the system of foodstuffs altered by means of high temperature, and by complicated treatments of ordinary products produced by nature.

2. *After the consumption of fresh raw foodstuffs, produced by nature, our blood formula does not change in any lapse of time, nor in consequence of any combinations.*

3. *After the consumption of foodstuffs produced by nature, but altered by means of high temperature, an augmentation of the general number of white corpuscles takes place, but the correlation of percentage between them remains the same.*

4. *After the consumption of foodstuffs produced by nature, but altered by manufacturing processes, an augmentation of the general number of white corpuscles as well as a change in the correlation of their percentage takes place.*

5. *It has been proved possible to take, without changing the blood formula, every kind of foodstuff which is habitually eaten now, but only by following this rule, viz: — that it must be taken along with raw products, according to a definite formula.*

6. *In a healthy organism, it is not possible, by the consumption of any food to alter the correlation of percentage between the white corpuscles, without augmenting their general number.*

7. *Foodstuffs do not seem to have any influence on the transitional and the Polymorphonuclear Eosinophiles and the correlation of percentage*

193

between them is not altered.

8. *We can change our blood formula in the direction we desire by dieting accordingly.*

9. *Blood examination can only have significance as a diagnosis if it is made on an empty stomach.*

Here I would quote from an address given at the 'Invitation of the Youth Welfare Association' held in Sydney, Australia in October, 1967, by Dr. Ralph Bircher of Zurich, Switzerland:

"First of all let me state our foremost conclusion in decisive terms: when a higher level of health is sought *the greatest single factor contributing to it is natural food as it comes from the soil.*

"I do not put this forward as a proposition, but as a *conclusion.* I do not put this forward as a personal whim, but as a *scientific fact. It has to be experienced to be believed.*

"I am now going to show you a part of a documentary film which makes the effect of natural food visible. In 1937, at the Royal Free Hospital in London, under the direction of a doctor trained by Dr. Bircher-Benner, a dozen patients stricken with chronic rheumatoid arthritis and completely resistant to orthodox treatment, permitted themselves to be experimented upon to see exactly what raw food could do to alleviate their condition. All drugs were strictly excluded. As you well know, arthritis lends itself perfectly to registering improvements and relapses in a film, for the disease affects the joints and therefore the mobility. This particular film was chosen not because it was the best but because it was the most instructive. It deals with a 55-year-old lady who had been sick for 2½ years and bedridden for six weeks, a miserable human wreck completely dependent on two persons for all her needs. It is an example of chronic rheumatoid arthritis in the 5th phase, that is to say she has been already declared to be beyond all reasonable hope. Again, let me call attention to the fact that she was treated, if that is the right word, with the strictest raw diet during the first fortnight, and after that she was permitted to include some conservatively cooked food as well. Perhaps her illness was too far advanced for this diet. After all it was a 'burnt-out' case.

"There was the patient lying on the bed, in great pain, trying to lift, with so much effort, her poor arms and feet, but could not sit up or remain sitting when put in a sitting position. Her body looked emaciated and terribly undernourished in spite of all their efforts to feed her well. After six weeks no improvement was perceptible and some doctors saw no reason to go on with the case; there were *hopeful cases* needing their urgent attention. It was the patient herself who begged them to go on. She said, 'I feel it's coming!' How brave she was: we have much to learn from such people. In the seventh week there was pandemonium; terrible pains, high fever, headaches. It looked like a complete relapse, a crime! Should they stop the experiment? But they recognized it as a *curative crisis*. The patient had trust in them and held out. She had nothing to lose and everything to win. In fact the crisis was good news, improbable and unexpected good news. It told that the *self-curing* process, with which every human is endowed, was not, in her case, entirely burnt out, that the *Inner Doctor*, as Hippocrates called it, effected a resurrection and the fight could be won. Let me say emphatically and without fear of contradiction that it was the power of the food that brought this about. For this is evidenced by the fact that nothing else — neither drugs, nor physical treatments, were applied. Step by step, from then on, the patient regained her mobility, in spite of her so-called starvation diet as conventional people like to regard it. After a little over a year she could return to her home, able to help herself and do light household work. She followed Dr. Bircher-Benner's advice about diet, three quarters of which, and always raw food first, consisted of raw food. Ten years later, at 66, she was able to do some digging in the garden and to feel the joy of growing the very food she was to eat. . . .

"Now I must tell you how I personally explain the vitalising power of raw food. I consider it even more important than all the other things put together, more than all the vitamins, mineral salts, enzymes, trace minerals, chlorophyll, plant antibiotics and the whole caboodle of things. You may buy vitamins at the drug store but you cannot buy in this way the special qualities to be found fresh in raw foods. They do not yield to extraction and preservation. One may say that *raw food contains Sun Energy, stored in living plant cells unspoilt by wilting, heating or industrial processing.* . . .

"I will conclude with an account of some impressive results in nutritional research. Professor Karl Eimer of the Medical Department of the University of Marburg picked out in 1937 a number of outstanding sportsmen among his students and made them undergo a two weeks' training along conventional lines. When they reached total fitness he suddenly and without warning switched them over to pure raw food. There was no transistional period. For these athletes it meant a diet they were unaccustomed to, and it meant a reduction of protein intake from 100 grams to 50 grams. The conventional diet was, as you may guess, mainly animal, and the new diet was, of course, almost purely of vegetable protein. I suspect the good Professor expected a complete breakdown and a disastrous decline in their performance. But nothing of the sort happened. They grew stronger, speedier and more supple. Here was revealed the economy and efficiency-raising effect of raw food in metabolism. It was, you will agree, a *remarkable* result.

"Another experiment was carried out in 1951 by Dr. Kuratsune, now Head of the Medical Department of the University of Kyushu, Japan. This experiment was actually carried out on his wife and himself. He imitated the under-nourishment conditions of the Concentration Camp as far as food quantities were concerned: 22-30 grams of protein, 7½-8½ grams of fat, 164-207 grams of carbohydrates and only 729-826 calories per day per 70 kgrs of body weight instead of 2150 calories. The actual quantities were even lower but he related them to 70 kgrs in order to make comparison possible.

"This he did during three relatively extended periods: a) 120 days in Winter, b) 32 days in Summer, and c) 81 days in Spring. He accomplished this experiment while fully occupied with this professional work and while his young wife was occupied with the feeding of their baby as well as the housework. That was the importance of such an experiment: According to all information from the hunger-stricken regions and camps, the rapid onset of the dread hunger-disease was bound to come with the resultant breakdown of resistance to infection and with anaemia. But nothing of the sort happened. The participants, note that I do not call them patients, continued in good health and in good working condition during the said periods, and the young lady was better able to feed her infant. What is the reason for this? The answer must have to come to you immediately. The food, though grossly insufficient, was fresh and raw. It consisted of whole grain rice, soaked and shredded, greens and a little fruit. There was no animal protein whatever. But take note of this: during the third experiment Kuratsune switched over to cooked food, exactly the same food, but this time *cooked*. As a result the dreaded hunger-disease seized them; collapse, hunger-oedema occurred, only to disappear when he switched back again to the uncooked diet."

An interesting article appeared in the July, 1975, issue of the Executive Health news report which indicates that the truth is seeping through and that diet is a factor, if not the main factor, in the cause of arthritis.

In this issue they quote many authorities, such as Dr. William Kaufman, a Connecticut internist; E. C. Barton-Wright, a biochemist; W. A. Elliott, physician-in-charge of the Rheumatic Clinic of St. Alfege's Hospital, London; Dr. John M. Ellis, Chief of Medical Staff at Titus County Memorial Hospital, Mt. Pleasant, Texas; and, last but not least, the famed Dr. Roger J. Williams of the University of Texas. It seems that each of these eminent men has come up with something that indicates that nutrition is a factor in arthritis.

I would like to sum up this information by quoting from Dr. Roger J. Williams's book, 'Nutrition Against Disease: Environmental Prevention':

"While medical education has put a damper on experiments in which the nutrition of arthritics might have been studied and manipulated in an expert fashion, there is excellent reason for thinking that if this were done, sufferers could get real rather than palliative relief. *There is even a good possibility that individual arthritics will be able — if they are lucky and make intelligent trials — to hit upon particular nutrients or nutrient combinations which will bring results.*

"I certainly would not want to give the impression that the management of these diseases is simple. But I do reaffirm the dictum that nutrition should be tried first. On the basis of reports presently available, the items that certainly need to be considered are niacin (niacinamide), pantothenic acid, riboflavin, vitamin A, vitamin B6, vitamin C, magnesium, calcium, phosphate and other minerals. The objective is to feed *adequately* the cells that are involved in keeping the bones, joints, and muscles in healthy condition."

It seems to me that at last the medical fraternity is slowly but surely being forced to admit that diet can be, or even is, a factor in arthritis. After denying and fighting this truth for hundreds of years or maybe longer, it must be painful for the medical profession to now begin to see the light. It is a bitter pill to swallow.

I say, "Don't treat your arthritis . . . fight it in the early stages with a raw food diet when you first see the signs, when it can be readily corrected. And, if you maintain the proper quota of raw food in your diet, it will never bother you again."

I consider a raw food diet to be the simplest, the most realistic and the safest means of conquering arthritis.

CHAPTER 27

ONLY NATURE CAN CURE

I have long rejected and refused to use the word 'cure' . . . except, of course, in very limited instances. The reason that I give is clear and to the point. If you are suffering from a skin problem, an arthritic condition, a heart ailment or any one of many other conditions that affect the human body, the condition can be remedied or alleviated by undergoing certain changes or taking certain drugs or treatments and you can say that you are cured. However, as soon as you go back to your old habits or forget to take your medicine or such, the disease comes back. Therefore, in most cases the cure was not a cure but a delusion.

I might phrase it a bit differently and say that you can't cure a disease any more than you can cure hunger or thirst. You can satisfy hunger and you can satisfy thirst, but it's only temporary. You get hungry and thirsty again, so the cure is gone.

By the methods that I advocate, a proper diet and proper way of life, most people can readily get rid of the conditions that afflict them . . . from the simple conditions to the serious conditions. It is not hard to make them go away by following a strict regimen of either proper diet or fasting, but that does not mean a cure. As soon as one returns to his old habits and forgets about the practices and principles that caused the condition to go away or regress, the condition returns and sometimes with greater viciousness than before. Thus, you can readily understand why I object to and seldom use the word 'cure'.

This does not mean that I do not believe that conditions, including arthritis, can be cured because I definitely do believe that you can cure them if you will follow the natural way of life and stay with it . . . but the cure will stay with you only as long as you stay with that way of life.

I would like to quote a recent article that appeared in the National Enquirer, written by James Gregory:

"Actress Cloris Leachman says being a vegetarian improved her health — but almost wrecked her marriage.

" 'I credit my mother-in-law, Mabel Albertson, the actress, for telling me about a new and healthy way of life,' the 48-year-old Oscar winner told The Enquirer.

"But Cloris said her husband, globe-trotting producer George Englund, 'was concerned that we couldn't travel as a family if the children and I were vegetarians.'

" 'He thought it would be ridiculous — that the children would be strange little people who wouldn't eat anything but certain nuts or fruits or vegetables.'

" 'We almost got a divorce over it,' Cloris added.

"However, Englund soon was impressed by the health benefits of the vegetarian diet. 'Now our whole family enjoys healthy, colorful and appetizing meatless foods,' Cloris said.

"In an interview in Brentwood, California, the actress recalled that she faced a health crisis 15 years ago when she developed severe asthma and arthritis in the joints of her fingers and she could only get 3 or 4 hours' sleep a night.

" 'In addition, I had hay-fever.'

"Her mother-in-law, a practicing vegetarian, prescribed a fast — permitting Cloris to have only fresh orange juice, relieved by an occasional glass of carrot juice with tiny cubes of ripe avocado in it.

"Within four days, Cloris said, her arthritis, asthma and hay-fever had vanished.

" 'The fasting and the orange and carrot juices cleaned the toxins out of my system. And I was sleeping well again.'

"Since then, Cloris has never eaten meat. She also tries to avoid such things as eggs, butter, milk, white bread and sugar.

"Cloris has no objection to being ridiculed for her diet of fruits and vegetables. She explained: 'Let them laugh, I say. We'll see who has the last laugh.' "

Here I must state what I consider to be an important bit of information. It has been proven that a cooked vegetable diet is no more beneficial or healthful to the human anatomy than a cooked carnivorous diet. In fact, evidence reveals that meat loses less in cooking than do vegetables. A raw vegetarian diet? Ah, that is an entirely different story! All the nutrients in a raw vegetable diet are available to your body to maintain it in good health.

Now I would like to quote something that appeared in a bulletin issued by The Arthritis Foundation, New Jersey Chapter, 26 Prospect St., Westfield, N.J. 07090, under the heading, "A Cure or a 'Happening'?":

"The Arthritis Foundation has been searching for a cure for arthritis for over 25 years. Yet, quacks all over the world are still talking about the 'cures' they offer. Maybe it is time to review the difference between a CURE and a HAPPENING.

"When medical science talks about a CURE, it means something more than just a temporary disappearance of symptoms. A temporary disappearance of symptoms cannot be considered a 'cure.' Such a condition is generally known as a 'spontaneous remission of symptoms,' which means that for some unknown reason the pain, discomfort or disability just happened to stop. With arthritis, remissions are not unusual; the average arthritis patient will experience remissions during the course of this disease.

"A medical CURE is a treatment which has a predictable effect and *works the same way against the same disease every time*. An example is the way certain antibiotics are a cure for pneumonia with a statistical certainty.

"The drugs, nostrums and gadgets that quacks claim as 'cures' do not act this way. Where they work at all, it is on a hit-or-miss basis. Most of their remedies gained their first claim as a 'cure' because some person used them just before a spontaneous remission was (for some unknown reason) due to occur. So, naturally, when the symptoms disappeared, the quack's 'miracle cure' received all of the credit.

"Be assured that when a real CURE for arthritis has been discovered and approved, it will receive worldwide publicity and will be available for everyone. It certainly will NOT be something that is 'secretly administered in a back room' or something that one will have to cross international borders to get."

Well, when the Arthritis Foundation talks about medical science bringing forth cures, this has just got to be the biggest laugh in history. However, it is not such a big joke to those who suffer from arthritis, for which the medical profession and the Arthritis Foundation have not as yet found a cure.

Please note, with emphasis, that the Arthritis Foundation mentions ONLY pneumonia. The AMA cannot cure a cold, asthma, heart disease, emphysema, cancer, arthritis or acne. In fact, the Arthritis Foundation mentioned about the only disease on the calendar that medical science can cure.

Yes, and even the cure for pneumonia, which is by means of antibiotics (penicillin, etc.) leaves the patient susceptible to any or all the other diseases and they are lucky if they do not succumb to one of these other diseases before they are many years older.

Now for the benefit of my readers and to contradict the Arthritis Foundation, the raw food diet that I advocate is not secretly administered and is not sold or bartered for . . . nor is there any fee of any kind involved.

There is a cure for arthritis and there has always been a cure for arthritis, but it is not in the best interests of the Arthritis Foundation or the American Medical Association to do research along the raw food diet lines. Both of these organizations, as you can readily understand, have just too much to lose and, therefore, they will never take the risk of supporting a completely raw food diet experiment.

In this selfsame bulletin from the Arthritis Foundation, there appeared the following notice:

"A bequest from the estate of Gay Weaver Illg has been received in the amount of $2,220.59.

"A bequest from the estate of Florence Fream has been received in the amount of $47,415.23."

And then they go on to tell you, under the heading "Memorials":

"A memorial gift to the Arthritis Foundation is a thoughtful tribute to the memory of a loved one — relative or friend. Such gifts serve the living through advancing medical research and education.

"Acknowledgments of memorials are always mailed the same day as received to both the bereaved and the donor.

"During 1973, the Chapter is most grateful to have received $7,572 from individuals, clubs and employee groups in memory of family or friends who have suffered with arthritis."

I am quoting this so that you will readily understand that I know what I am saying and I want you to know, too, so that you can better understand why no cure for arthritis is forthcoming now or ever from the AMA or the Arthritis Foundation. Furthermore, now you can better understand why they ridicule those who have had any part in defeating arthritis and in bringing forth testimonials from those who actually were cured.

Another bit of interesting information about these foundations. There used to be the National Foundation for Infantile Paralysis and then it shifted to birth defects and arthritis . . . probably because the money for polio dried up and they didn't want to be left out in the cold.

Here I would like to quote this story from the book, "The Doctors' Dilemmas," by Louis Lasagna, M.D.:

"In 1958, having 'solved' the polio problem, the National Foundation for Infantile Paralysis broadened its scope, in an attempt to perpetuate its fund-raising activities. The name was changed to the National Foundation, and the emphasis shifted to birth defects and arthritis. The move brought the NF into direct conflict with the already existent Arthritis and Rheumatism Foundation. Merger talks — allegedly initiated by the ARF — resulted in an offer from Basil O'Connor, first and only president of the NF, to absorb the ARF into the larger NF structure. The Arthritis Foundation refused, issuing a statement in which they asked the National Foundation to hold off its entry into the arthritis field for one year, to see whether the '10,000,000 sufferers from arthritis . . . need more than one foundation working in the same field.' The polio people retorted that 'individual diseases are not the personal property of individual organizations' and plunged in, providing what some consider to be an unneeded duplication of activities in the arthritis field, but what others consider an important extra shot in the arm for rheumatology."

There you have a little bit of the true story concerning the many money collecting organizations, the Arthritis Foundation and others. And now you know why they have not found a cure and never will find a cure for arthritis.

As the title of this chapter says, "Only nature can cure!"

CHAPTER 28

QUESTIONS AND ANSWERS

Here I will give you my answers to some of the most frequently asked questions on arthritis.

Q. *Can I defeat arthritis by myself, without the aid of a doctor of any kind?*

A. Why would you need a doctor to embark on a raw food diet? For the first time in your life you will be following biological law and doing something really worthwhile for your health. On the other hand, if you feel that a healer is necessary, then by all means go to one. I say to rely on your own intelligence, your own will power and your own intuition.

Q. *Do you advocate that we eat raw meat, raw fish and raw eggs?*

A. Why not? All carnivorous animals who consume such commodities raw seem to fare quite well. However, I do not advocate a carnivorous diet, I suggest a diet of raw vegetables, grains, fruits and nuts.

Q. *How long will it take to get results from a raw food diet?*

A. I presume you want me to tell you that it will only take a couple of days to get results with a raw food diet. Well, it's not quite that way! Remember, it took anywhere from 10 to 50 years to develop the condition from which you are suffering. However, I will tell you that ten days will give you an inkling as to the benefits and thirty days will show you the light and give you every indication of definite improvement. Then from thirty days on, the results will be so manifest that you will never change for the rest of your life.

Q. *Will the sudden change of diet cause any stomach problems?*

A. I always warn that it sometimes takes up to two weeks for the body to adjust to the drastic changes that take place on the raw food diet. Yes, and it is even longer for some people. You may have a bit of discomfort here and there or a bit of diarrhea during the first two weeks but after that you should have no problems whatsoever.

Q. *Do I need vitamins and food supplements to assist me in gaining good health and freedom from arthritis?*

A. Get your vitamins from raw vegetables, grains, fruits and nuts. There is no vitamin pill or food supplement on earth that even remotely compares in value to the healing power and health-giving properties of a raw food diet composed of mainly raw vegetables, some grains, some fruits and a few nuts. However, if you feel good natural vitamins will help — by all means, use them.

Q. *Why do you insist upon a raw food diet in the treatment of arthritis?*

A. A famed Swiss medical doctor proved conclusively and without a shadow of doubt that all cooked foods are toxic to the human body. Those who eat mostly cooked food in their regular diet suffer the most and those who eat less cooked food suffer less.

Q. *I am a busy man and I cannot afford the time it takes to get all the vegetables, the time it takes to prepare them and the time it takes to chew and digest them. Can't I eat conventional cooked food and supplement my diet with vitamin pills?*

A. If you don't take the time to live, you will soon have to take the time to die. There is no man or woman alive in America today who cannot take enough time off to eat at least one big vegetable salad each day.

Q. *I take vitamins because I was told that the land on which we grow our vegetables is depleted and does not contain adequate quantities of the essential vitamins and minerals. Is that so?*

A. If raw natural foods no longer contain the essential nutrients, then where in heaven's name would the vitamin manufacturers get them? I suggest that even supermarket vegetables contain a good supply of fairly well balanced nutrients. Besides, most vitamin tablets are synthetic, no matter what their makers claim, so you can't expect to find your minerals and vitamins in these pills. However, I suppose that taking vitamins and food supplements is better than doing nothing.

Q. *Are herbal remedies reliable or worthwhile in the treatment of arthritis?*

A. Having studied the results of herbalism for many years, I feel that it is virtually impossible to do harm with the proper use of herbs. Further, the herbal practitioner and various other individuals who have used herbs for

211

arthritis do claim a high rate of benefits and cures. Personally, I would trust properly administered herbs and a qualified herbalist before drugs and surgery.

Q. *I hear and read of people who have suffered from arthritis and gained a spontaneous remission by the laying on of hands. What can you tell me about this?*

A. People who practise the laying on of hands — Kathryn Kuhlman, Oral Roberts, Harry Edwards and many others — believe that this happens. However, and get this straight, there are still millions of Americans suffering the pain, discomfort and agony of arthritis, so don't count on a spontaneous remission . . . unearned. Still I see no risk or harm in seeking help through this medium.

Q. *Surely, Mr. Tobe, you are aware that a totally raw food diet is virtually impossible or at least impractical for the average person. Can't you be a little more merciful and strike a compromise somewhere along the line?*

A. Yes, you are right. A totally raw food diet is difficult or well nigh impossible for the average American. However, I am not playing God, so it is not for me to have mercy. I insist on a completely raw food diet whenever possible because experience has taught me that if a little leeway is given, the backsliding begins and grows . . . to nullify the effect.

Q. *Do you mean to suggest that the medical profession is wrong and you are right?*

A. It is not I who is right . . . it is nature. I am stating clearly and emphatically to all who will listen that only nature can heal.

Q. *Does climate affect arthritis? A friend of mine told me that if I moved to a dry climate such as Arizona I would definitely get relief from my arthritis.*

A. Some people claim that warmth does give them some comfort and some relief but my reading and investigations reveal that heat or a change in climate will not result in a cure or even a betterment in the arthritic condition. If climate were a factor in arthritis, then Arizona and New Mexico would have an influx of probably 20,000,000 or 30,000,000 arthritic sufferers from all parts of America. My advice is to stay where you are but change your eating and living habits.

Q. *Why do more women than men suffer from arthritis?*

A. This is a very difficult question and I am afraid I do not have a definite answer. I have always maintained that women eat more greens and salads than men and if this is so, then women should suffer less from arthritis than men. However, facts are facts and more women suffer from arthritis than men.

Perhaps the reason lies in the fact that most housewives indulge in their cup of tea or coffee or other boiled beverage, when at home or out visiting, more often than men.

It is generally recognized that in osteoporosis the percentage of women runs about four times as high as men. Women have been given hormonal shots and drugs for well over 25 years and it is suspected that the use of hormones is a major contributing factor in the cause of osteoporosis. The menses may also be one of the reasons why women are more prone to this condition.

Q, *Is salt a contributor to arthritis?*

A. It has long been my belief that salt contributes to many diseases that afflict man since it is known to impair or interfere with the function of many of the organs of the

213

body. Yes, I would consider salt a factor in the cause of arthritis.

Q. *Is a heavy protein diet a factor in arthritis?*

A. I would heartily agree that a heavy protein diet can and does contribute to arthritis. In fact, it could also contribute to many other diseases, including cancer. If the protein in your diet is derived from whole foods such as vegetables, grains and nuts, then there is never any danger of getting too high a protein content in your diet. However, those who are heavy meat and fish eaters will run into difficulties because of the lack of adequate carbohydrate. While as of this moment I have no conclusive proof, I would say that a high protein diet could very well be a factor in the cause of arthritis.

Q. *Do X-rays cause arthritis?*

A. X-rays are involved in so many conditions and diseases that they surely must be a contributing factor in arthritis. Anyone who will take the time and the trouble to investigate will find that there is no safe threshold level with X-rays. Whether the X-ray involved is of a tooth or an extremity or any other part of your body, each X-ray does cause damage. Therefore, there is no question whatsoever, X-rays play a role in the cause of arthritis. The more X-rays you have, the more you will suffer from arthritis or other conditions.

The insidious part of this X-ray business is the fact that the effects of X-rays take months and often years to become apparent. Thus, because of the passing of time, seldom is the X-ray blamed. In general, the medical profession prefers to ignore the fact that the X-ray might be and probably is the guilty culprit in many unexplained diseases.

Q. *I was told that if I ate more than ten percent of my diet in raw foods, I could avoid or get rid of arthritis. Is this true?*

A. I wish it were that simple. There is no doubt about it, the average American diet does not contain 10% raw food and, therefore, 10% would at least be a step in the right direction. The way I prefer to phrase it is that you will get rid of arthritis in proportion to the amount of raw food in your diet. If you want to be sure and safe, a totally raw food diet is the safest and surest way to avoid arthritis or rid yourself of arthritis and regain your normal health.

Q. *Why is arthritis striking so many young people today?*

A. Well, I have a couple of reasons that could be an important consideration in this. First and foremost, children from 3 and 4 years of age are taught to eat hamburgers, hotdogs, French fries and soda pop, none of which could by any stretch of the imagination be construed as raw food.

When I was a youngster, we ate an apple, a banana or maybe a pear or a peach as a snack but today instead of this children eat hotdogs, hamburgs and French fries, all of which contribute to arthritis and other diseases.

The second reason as I see it, is that most infants do not get their start in life on mother's milk. Breast feeding is the proper way to raise an infant and breast feeding for the first year or two of the child's life gives him an exceptionally good start.

Today it is a rarity to find a child who is reared from the breast. Instead, they usually get a formula of cow's milk which is of course heated and treated and contains no enzymes. Therefore, they do not get a proper start in life.

Q. *Why do doctors so very often prescribe cortisone or other corticosteroids?*

A. There are a few reasons why doctors will prescribe these deadly, dangerous drugs. The first could be that the patient is suffering greatly and actually demands that the doctor give him something to relieve the pain. Cortisone and its derivitives can perform that function. But almost invariably there will be serious side effects ... much more serious than the original arthritis or other conditions.

However, a patient who is in agony or suffering is not very concerned with what will happen to him in 2 or 3 or 5 or more years. So I assume that the medical doctor weighs the matter in the balance and makes the decision on the basis of his patient's wishes.

Another reason that many doctors prescribe the cortisone type drugs is because they do in most cases give prompt relief and mask the symptoms and the doctor receives credit for this miracle. Many doctors don't worry about what is going to happen to the patient in 2 or 3 or 5 years.

Q. *Do you know of any specific cases where a raw food diet has actually performed the miracle of making a crippled person walk again?*

A. Yes, there are many on record if you will bother to investigate but a prime example is that of a friend of mine, Rear-Admiral Al Malstrom, United States Navy (Ret'd) who received the best attention that the American government could provide and he was sentenced to spend the rest of his life in a wheelchair in Walter Reed Hospital.

However, he heard of the virtues of raw food and tried it and today he is a perfect specimen of man and today his diet is — you guessed it — all raw food. He is a peripatetic purveyor of what proper nutrition can do for a man.

Q. *I have heard of success with potato and onion or flaxseed poultices applied to the affected parts of the body for the relief of arthritis. What is your opinion?*

A. I do not laugh at any of these so-called natural remedies. I tell of many methods that are used throughout the world. They may seem strange or unusual and some even sound ridiculous but some people insist that they have brought help and results and perhaps a remission. In my opinion the poultice of onions and potatoes or flax is certainly to be preferred over aspirin, the cortisone type of drug, surgery, X-ray or radium.

Q. *Should I take regular exercise for my arthritis or would it be better if I rested more?*

A. I strongly recommend as much exercise as possible. As a young man I learned a little rhyme that said, "If you rest, you rust and if you rust you will bust."
I agree that rest is essential for health and long life but too much rest is perhaps as bad or worse than not enough. By all means, exercise within reason. Get as much exercise as your body can tolerate.

BIBLIOGRAPHY

VOLUMES, BOOKS, BOOKLETS

1. The Merck Index, Seventh and Eleventh Editions
2. Chamber's Dictionary of Science and Technology
3. Davidson's Principles and Practice of Medicine
4. Taber's Cyclopedic Medical Dictionary
5. The Vitamins in Medicine — *Franklin Bicknell, D.M., M.R.C.P. and Frederick Prescott, M.Sc., Ph.D., A.R.I.C., M.R.C.S.*
6. Vitamin and Mineral Therapy — *Funk and Dubin*
7. Uncooked Foods — *Eugene Christian*
8. The Vitamins and Their Clinical Application — *Stepp, Kuhnau, Schroeder*
9. A Dictionary of Biology — *Abercrombie, Hickman, Johnson*
10. Nutrition Against Disease — *Roger J. Williams, M.D.*
11. There Is a Cure For Arthritis — *Paavo Airola*
12. New Hope For Arthritis Sufferers — *Max Warmbrand, N.D., D.O.*
13. Get Well Naturally — *Linda Clark*
14. The Arthritis Cook Book — *Dong and Banks*
15. Dr. Bircher-Benner's Way to Positive Health and Vitality
16. The Elixir of Life — *Arnold DeVries*

17. Banish Arthritis — *Rudolph*
18. Living With Arthritis — *Dr. A. B. Corrigan*
19. Arthritis — *MacFarlane*
20. Arthritis and Rheumatism — *Weger, Tilden, Fleming*
21. Rheumatism and Arthritis — *Editorial Committee, Science of Life Books*
22. Suggestions for the Arthritic — *Lager and Jones*
23. Beneficial Effects of Whole Body Internal Irradiation — *Lewis*
24. Therapeutic Fasting — *Paavo Airola*
25. Arthritis and Folk Medicine — *D. C. Jarvis, M.D.*
26. How Thousands of My Arthritis Patients Regained Their Health — *Max Warmbrand, N.D., D.O.*
27. Arthritis Can Be Cured — *Bernard Aschner, M.D.*
28. The Fountain of Youth — *Arnold DeVries*
29. A Doctor's Proven New Home Cure for Arthritis — *Campbell*
30. Arthritis and Common Sense — *Alexander*
31. Arthritis, Rheumatism and Your Aching Back — *J. I. Rodale*
32. The Arthritis Handbook — *Crain*
33. Overcoming Rheumatism and Arthritis — *Speight*
34. Sciatica — *Bohun-Greene*
35. Why Suffer Needless Arthritis and Bursitis Pain? — *Sides*
36. The Doctors' Dilemmas — *Louis Lasagna, M.D.*
37. Arthritis Basic Facts — *The Arthritis Foundation*
38. There's Help For Arthritis — *LaRue Stone and Lawrence E. Lamb, M.D.*
39. Arthritis and Radioactivity — *Lewis*
40. Overcoming Arthritis and Rheumatism — *Jensen*
41. Applied Trophology — *Various Authors*
42. The Complete Book of Food and Nutrition — *J. I. Rodale*

43. The Vitamins — *A Symposium*
44. Vitamins, A Survey of Present Knowledge — *Medical Research Council (G.B.)*
45. Clinical Toxicology of Commercial Products — *Gleason, etc.*
46. When Doctors Are Patients — *Pinner and Miller*
47. The Complete Book of Vitamins — *J. I. Rodale*
48. Arthritis and Rheumatism — *Walter C. Alvarez, M.D.*
    Newspaper Reports
    Research Papers
    Magazine Articles

Index

A

Adrenocortical steroids, 160
Advertising, 24
Airola, Dr. Paavo, 20
Alfalfa, 148, 171
Alka butazolidin, 178
Almquist and Stokstad, 68
Alvarez, Dr. Walter C., 6
American Journal of Clinical Nutrition, 74
Analgesia, 156
Animals, 5, 18
Antiarthritics, 162
Antigout, 163
Antimalarial drugs, 15
Arthritis Foundation, 11, 20, 97, 174, 203
Arthritis philosophy, 1
Arthritis psychology, 1
Arthroclasia, 92
Arthrodesis, 92
Arthroplasty, 92
Aspirin, 12, 14, 26, 69, 115, 156, 168, 173, 176
Atrophic arthritis, 19

B

Bad Gastein Mine, 131
Bed rest, 84
Behaviour modification therapy, 3
Benson E. F., 165
Beverages, 63
Bicknell and Prescott, 41, 45, 52, 120, 139
Biopsies, 93

Bircher, Dr. Ralph, 194
Blistering plasters, 153
Blood formula, 193
Bonica, Dr. John J., 20, 80
Bread, 57
Bruce's Materia Medica, 118
Bursitis, 8, 19, 65

C

Calcium, 34, 47, 52, 74
Cancer, 16, 17, 99, 109, 135, 140
Carotene, 42
Cataract, 16
Causes, 21, 31
Cellular regeneration process, 18
Certo, 170
Charcot's joint, 19
Charnley, Dr. John, 96, 100
Chelates, 173
Chiropractors, 103
Chloroquine, 158
Cholecalciferol, 54
Cider vinegar, 143
Clark, Linda, 184
Cleave, Dr. T. L., 60
Climate, 212
Codeine, 155
Cod liver oil, 52, 137
Concentrated foods, 60
Contraction release, 92
Cooked food, 31, 39, 68
Copper, 172, 173
Cornell University Arthritis Clinic, 71
Corrigan, Dr. A. B., 11
Corticosteroids, 155, 158, 160, 161, 216

Corticotropin, 132
Cortisone, 16, 26, 32, 83, 132, 176, 216
Cosmetics, 47
Counterirritants, 156
Critical temperature, 191
Cure, 201

D

Dairy products, 31, 46
Dam, Pro. Henrik, 138
Darley, Dr. Robert, 52
Dermatitis, 158
DeVries, Arnold, 20, 21
Dexamethasone, 160
Dicumarol, 120
Diet, 9, 18, 40, 128, 153, 164, 182, 185, 195, 201
Dimercaprol, 158
Drugs, 33, 34, 78
Drying food, 69

E

Eimer, Prof. Karl, 196
Emotion, 71
Emotional problems, 32
Empirin compound, 155
Enzymes, 31, 37, 65, 144
Enzyme-engineering, 37
Eosinophiles, 193
Eosinophilia, 157
Episiotomy, 117
Essential unsaturated fatty acids, 41
Executive Health, 198
Exercise, 31, 34, 85, 161, 217

F

Fabry's disease, 37
Family dynamics, 3

Family Health Magazine, 93
Fasting, 123, 153
Fibromyositis, 19
Fibrositis, 7
Fish, 46
Food supplements, 210
Frozen foods, 67

G

Galen, 155
Gaucher's disease, 37
Geometric total knee surgery, 97
Gold compound, 156, 157
Gold salts, 15
Gout, 8, 19, 37
Grains, 47
Grossman, Dr. Morton I., 116

H

Hare, Dorothy C., C.B.E., M.D., 185
Heart disease, 41
Heating of foods, 34
Heberden's nodes, 8
Helmer and Jansen, 46
Hematogenous metastatic infection, 100
Hemopoietic toxicity, 158
Hench, Dr. Philip, 8
Henn, Dr. Otto, 131
Herbal remedies, 211
Hippocratic Oath, 11
Honey, 143
Human milk, 49
Huebner and Link, 120
Hunter-Hurler syndrome, 38
Hyalex, 162
Hydrarthrosis, 19
Hydrochloric acid, 74
Hydrocortisone acetate, 160

Hydrocortisone tertiary-butylacetate, 160
Hydrogenated oil, 55
Hydrogenation, 42
Hydroxychloroquine, 155
Hypertrophic arthritis, 19
Hypoprothrombinaemia, 69, 120

I

Iatrogenic diseases, 83
Iatrogeny, 84
Ibuprofen, 117, 168
Indomethacin, 15, 118, 156, 158, 176
Infectious arthritis, 8, 19
Intra-articular hormonal treatment, 161

J

Jarvis, Dr. D.C., 143
Journal of the American Medical Association, 116, 120, 131

K

Katz, Dr. Ronald, 79
Keller, Dr. W. D., 64
Kornbleuh, Igho Hart, M.D., 132
Kouchakoff, Paul, M.D., 31, 189
Kuroda, Paul K., Ph.D., 132

L

Lamb, Lawrence E., M.D., 10
Lasagna, Louis, M.D., 206
Lewis, John T., 130, 134
Lewis, Wade V., 130

Liniments, 79
Liposomes, 38
Lymphocytes, 175

M

Maleev, Dr. Atanas, 117
Marie-Strumpell arthritis, 19
Margarine, 55
Markolf, Dr. Keith, 99
Masseurs, 104
McMaster University, 3
Medical code, 24
Medical Letter, The, 108, 117
Medical Post, 97, 98, 99, 178
Merck Index, 120
Meyer and Howard, 120
Miami Herald, 178
Milk, 34, 46, 74
Mineral baths, 129
Mineral oil, 55, 70
Motrin, 178
Muscular dystrophy, 139, 142
Myositis, 19

N

National Enquirer, 202
National Foundation, 206
Natural foods, 39
Neoplasms of joints, 8
Neuritis, 8
Neurogenic arthropathy, 19
News and World Report, The, 121
Niemann-Pick disease, 38
Nutrition, 34, 156, 198
Nutritional Review, 116

O

O'Brien, Robert, 132
Oils, 33, 42

Ormandy, Eugene, 93
Osteoarthritis, 16, 17, 19, 93, 117
Osteomalacia, 51
Osteoporosis, 213
Osteotomy, 92
Oxidative rancidity, 42

P

Pain, 77, 153, 156
Paracelsus, 153
Paracentesis, 161
Pasteurization, 34
Paulus, Dr. Harold, 175
Percival, Dr. Thomas, 52
Peter, Dr. James, 175
Phenylbutazone, 15, 155, 158, 168
Phosphate, 54
Phosphorus, 47, 52
Physiotherapy, 161
Poison oak, 171
Poisoned environment, 34
Pompe's disease, 38
Pottenger, Dr. Francis, 35
Prednizolone, 160
Processed food, 31, 39
Proliferative arthritis, 19
Prosthesis, 96
Prosthetic replacement parts, 28
Protein, 214
Prothrombin, 67, 119
Pruritis, 158
Psoriasis, 8
Psychogenic rheumatism, 8
Purging, 154

Q

Quacks, 9
Quick, A. J., 67

R

Rancid fats, 139
Raw food, 9, 18, 40, 128, 153, 181, 205, 209
Raw potato, 168
Rawls, W.B., 69
Reader's Digest, 132
Reesman, A. L., 65
Refined food, 34, 39
Rest, 156
Rheumatic fever, 8, 19, 120
Rheumatism, 7, 52
Rheumatoid arthritis, 6, 8, 10, 15, 16, 19, 37, 69, 89, 117, 131, 156, 158, 162, 174, 194
Rickets, 45, 48, 51
Rodale, J.I., 118
Roth, Dr. James, 119
Roughage, 59

S

Salicylates, 156
Salt, 22, 33, 213
Schroeder, Henry A., M.D., 60
Sciatica, 8
Science Digest, 163
Science News, 37
Scott, Cyril, 147
Scully, Francis J., M.D., 131
Sea water, 169
Seeds, 41, 47
Self-help devices, 28, 162
Selye, Prof. Hans, 73
Senescent arthritis, 8, 19
Sex, 111
Shelton, Dr. Herbert M., 124, 127
Shock treatment, 162
Shouldice Clinic, 84

Side effects, 15, 26, 84, 155, 158
Sinclair, Dr. Hugh N., 41
Sisk, Dr. Charles W., 175
Sleep, 29
Slipped disc, 8
Soaps, 47
Sodium salicylate, 156
Sorenson, Dr. John R. J., 173
Spas, 129
Spondylitis, 8, 19, 65
Spurs, 65
Steroids, 16, 160, 168, 176
Still's disease, 19
Stiner, Dr. O., 184
Stone, LaRue, 10
Stress, 73
Sugar, 33
Sulfa drugs, 70
Supplements, 53
Surgery, 28, 91, 105, 161, 176
Surgeyev, Dr. S. I., 99
Synovectomy, 92
Synovial fluid, 22, 95
Synovial membrane, 161
Synovioma, 19
Synovitis, 160
Syringomyelia, 19

T

Taber's Cyclopedic Medical Dictionary, 83
Tabes dorsalis, 19
Tay-Sachs disease, 38
Thyroid, 119
Time Magazine, 101
Tocopherols, 139
Total hip operation, 96
Toxemia, 22
Trace minerals, 60
Traction, 107
Trauma, 19
Tregilgas, Harold R., M.D., 130

U

Uranium-Radon Mine, 130
U.S. Dept. of Agriculture, 34
U.S. News & World Report, 48
U.S.S.R., 163

V

Van Dellen, T. R., M.D., 167
Vegetarian, 202
Vinegar, 143
Violet leaves, 168
Vitamins, 210
Vitamin A, 42
Vitamin B, 31, 42
Vitamin C, 21, 31, 74, 116
Vitamin D, 31, 45, 137, 140
Vitamin E, 31, 42, 139, 142
Vitamin F, 41
Vitamin K, 67, 120

W

Warmbrand, Max, N.D., D.O., 20
Water, 64
Weber, H., 108
Weissmann, Gerald, 37
Wheat products, 57
White, Dr. Paul Dudley, 116
White blood cells, 175
White corpuscles, 189
Wilde, Dr. Alan H., 94, 98
Williams, Dr. Roger J., 198
Wills, M. R., 53
Wilson, Dr. Philip, 100
World Congress of Gastroenterology, ll6

XYZ

X-rays, 29, 108, 161, 214
Young Arthritics in Action, 12